SOURCEBOOK FOR APHASIA

SOURCEBOOK FOR APHASIA
A GUIDE TO FAMILY ACTIVITIES
AND COMMUNITY RESOURCES

SUSAN HOWELL BRUBAKER, M.S., CCC-SP
Speech and Language Pathology Department
William Beaumont Hospital
Royal Oak, Michigan

Introductions by MICHAEL I. ROLNICK, Ph.D.

Wayne State University Press   Detroit 1982

Library of Congress Cataloging in Publication Data

Brubaker, Susan Howell, 1949–
  Sourcebook for aphasia.

  Bibliography: p.
  1. Aphasics—Rehabilitation—Problems, exercises,
etc. 2. Community health services. I. Title.
RC425.B778   616.85'5206   81-23099
ISBN 0-8143-1697-2 (pbk.)   AACR2

This publication is made possible in part through a grant from the
Village Woman's Club of Bloomfield Hills, Michigan, and The Goad
Foundation, in memory of Louis Clifford Goad.

To Ellen Watson Howell

CONTENTS

ACKNOWLEDGMENTS

The author would like to thank Cheryl Hutton, Carolyn Starrett, and Patricia Wierzbicki for their help with typing the manuscript; to Geraldine Dunkle for help with proofreading; to the Village Woman's Club of Bloomfield Hills, Michigan; The Goad Foundation; and especially to Clarissa Adams Goad for her support and suggestions.

MESSAGE TO THE CLINICIAN

The intent of this message is to help you become familiar with the contents of this book, whose format is unique to aphasia treatment. This book is partly didactic, partly informational, and partly therapeutic. It was written for the families of aphasic patients, for their use under your guidance. It is appropriate for any level patient. The type and severity of aphasia makes no difference since you will be individualizing the activities for each patient.

This book was conceived to remedy two major frustrations of aphasiologists. The first is the difficulty of getting the family involved in the rehabilitation process in an organized fashion. Carryover of treatment has always been a problem, and telling or showing someone how to work with the aphasic person can sometimes get no further than the treatment-room door. It is also important for the family members to know at what level their loved one is functioning. By working with the patient on some of the activities (see Section I) the family will have a much better idea of what aphasia involves and how recovery is proceeding. Although practice does not necessarily make perfect in dealing with aphasia, it certainly has its merits. It is hoped that these activities will stimulate carryover from formal treatment sessions. Perhaps the patient will become more involved in his own rehabilitation if part of his daily routine includes a variety of activities, games, and interactions. Patients also enjoy having a book, or other tangible item of their own—something to be used, shown to others, and referred to.

The second major frustration that this book attempts to remedy is the lack of answers to important family questions. Often we are not able to anticipate family problems or immediately find sources of information when needed. A well-intentioned family may be totally at a loss. They may not have any idea of what they need, or what might be worth exploring. In general, the process of family education and adjustment is an important part of rehabilitation. The intent, then, is for each family to have this book as a reference source and to use it under the clinician's guidance as an adjunct to formal treatment sessions. Throughout the book, there are many opportunities for you to make notes for the patient, add to the listings given, or make other comments.

The following explanations will give you an overview of the book and its intended usage.

SECTION I: ACTIVITIES. This is the longest section and the one which you will individualize and direct for the patient. The activities are divided into eleven general areas of possible impairment. They can be used separately or in combination, depending on communicative difficulties. Each activity has a place for you to check whether it is to be practiced by the patient. The first page of each of the eleven areas has a portion for you to fill out indicating how you want the family member to work with the patient (length of time, number of sessions, how to handle errors, and whether he is to also look for activities in other areas). These activities are not meant as a therapy "cookbook" but as additional practice for skills which the patient is developing in formal treatment. Caution the family to try only those activities which you have checked. Space has been designated at the beginning of each of the eleven areas as well as at the end for you to add any notes or special instructions. You will find that the activities take a minimum of preparation time and use only those materials likely to be available in a home or hospital. The progression of activities is generally from simple to more difficult. There are a few exceptions within the eleven areas when a different track is undertaken, such as reading comprehension versus reading aloud. Four appendixes list examples of items needed for certain activities and how to make or find them.

SECTION II: GAMES AND OTHER PASTIMES. This section focuses on patient and family interaction. All of the items here have been screened for aphasic use and are therefore recommended. Each one is annotated to indicate basic skills needed before it should be used with the patient. The games were picked because of their easy availability at most stores. You might want to suggest certain games which you think would be better than others, based on knowledge of your patient. **Solitaire Games** and **Things To Do Alone** are important for a patient's development so that he is not always dependent on someone else for his amusement. There is also space reserved for you to make notes in this section.

SECTION III: COMMUNITY RESOURCES. Often the patient and/or family need information or help, but do not know how to start, who to contact, or where to go. This section addresses these concerns. The eleven divisions represent areas most frequently asked about by patients and their families. Many possible sources of information or help have been suggested and explained. Space has also been reserved on the right side of each page for notation.

SECTION IV: SUGGESTED READING LIST. More than ninety publications were reviewed, and those chosen were thought to be most appropriate for family members experiencing aphasia for the first time. Most selections are annotated. There is space for you to add other readings or suggestions.

The last two pages of the book are very important. They contain a book order form and a form to be used when new books, games, and resources are discovered by those who use this book (professionals as well as families and patients). As there will be updates to this publication, information must be current for it to be useful. Any input you can give for future printings will be appreciated.

MESSAGE TO THE FAMILY

This book is designed and written for you—members of the family of an aphasic adult. Although it is meant to be used with the guidance of your speech-language pathologist, it is also your book to use as you please.

The sections of this book are very different. It is suggested that you read the entire book in order to get the most from it. Helpful ideas may be found where you least expect them. You may want to mark important items so that you can refer back to them at another time.

Each patient's aphasia varies; however, there are many similarities regardless of how mild or severe the resulting problems are. Therefore, even though your family member may have difficulties that seem much different from another person's, you can benefit from some of the same things and share some of the same frustrations. As you know, when someone in a family becomes aphasic, the changes and adjustments that affect the entire family are both subtle and obvious.

This book is divided into four major sections. The first section is an ACTIVITIES section to be used under the guidance of your speech-language pathologist. The second has suggestions for GAMES AND OTHER PASTIMES for the patient. The third section is on the COMMUNITY RESOURCES which can help you locate services in your area. The fourth section is a SUGGESTED READING LIST. Four appendixes are included for use with the Activities section.

It is important to realize that throughout the book the aphasic person is referred to as "he" or "the patient." The author is well aware that not all those with aphasia are males, but this seemed to be the best way to handle the dilemma. Your speech-language pathologist will also be referred to as "your clinician"—another title for the same person.

Finally, this is the kind of book which needs to be updated in order to be kept current. If you find something that is especially helpful and is not included in this edition, please share it with the author and others who will be using this book. Use the Suggestion Form at the back of the book for this purpose.

ACTIVITIES

Introduction

Family involvement during speech and language rehabilitation is important for successful treatment. No program can provide enough treatment to help the patient recover communicative skills without outside activities. In a true sense, then, helping a person recover from aphasia is a team approach. This section is designed to help you become part of that team.

In order to involve the family, this section presents a variety of activities which will be assigned by your speech-language pathologist. In this way the family can help reinforce treatment. It is important to remember that this does not teach you to become a clinician, but does open the door to many useful and beneficial ideas that will encourage communication. This joint effort will be most helpful in achieving rehabilitation goals.

All too often aphasic patients tend not to use their new speech and language skills at home because they fear failure. For this reason your clinician will select some activities that will be easiest for the patient to do during a particular point in his treatment. This will encourage him to participate with the family and practice speech and language skills.

Perhaps the most important result of helping your family member is the feeling of doing things together again. There is a danger, however. That danger is too much frustration. No activity should be continued if you or the patient become angry or frustrated. Care should be taken not to place too much pressure on him during these activities.

M. R.

How To Use the Activities

There are nearly 300 activities with suggestions for many more variations, simplifications, and expansions in this section of the book. These are divided among eleven areas of possible difficulties that the patient may be experiencing. You will not be doing all of them, just those which your speech-language pathologist feels are important, and these activities are indicated with a check mark.

At the beginning of each of the eleven areas, there is a paragraph or two explaining why those activities are together. There is also a list of specific instructions on how long to work at a session, whether or not to correct the patient if he makes a mistake, whether or not to keep track of errors, and whether to do several activities or only one at each working session.

When you find an activity that is checked, you will see that it has several parts to it. Let's take a look at each part separately so you will know how to read and understand them.

The activities are put together like this:

_____ ACTIVITY #:
MATERIALS:
WHAT TO DO:
EXAMPLE:
REMINDER:
VARIATION:
SIMPLIFYING THE ACTIVITY:
EXPANDING THE ACTIVITY:

The line _____ in front of the activity is there for the speech-language pathologist. If your clinician feels that the patient should practice this particular activity, he will put a check on that line. There may be checks for activities in any of the eleven areas.

ACTIVITY: The activities are numbered chronologically from 1 to 273. A few words describe what the activity is about.

MATERIALS: Any preparation or things that you will need in order to do the activity are stated here. Sometimes you will see this: (see Appendix). This refers to the appropriate appendix for suggestions as to where to find the necessary materials.

WHAT TO DO: The instructions for you to follow in the activity are explained here. They are written to whoever is doing the activity with the aphasic person. The patient is referred to as "he" whether the "he" is a male or female. This is much less awkward than he/she or him/her. Therefore, if it reads: "Say a word out loud" then it refers to you. If it says "he repeats it" then it refers to the aphasic patient. Your speech-language pathologist will be referred to as "your clinician" throughout this section of the book.

EXAMPLE: This provides a sample activity and tells how to do it.

REMINDER: This adds another idea to the main activity or emphasizes a special point if needed.

VARIATION: This suggests other ways to try the activity. You do not have to try the variation, but it is included if you would like a change.

SIMPLIFYING THE ACTIVITY: If the patient is having difficulty with the activity, or if his answers are wrong more than one-quarter of the time, then you should make the activity easier for him. This part will give you directions on how to simplify it.

EXPANDING THE ACTIVITY: If the activity is too easy for him or begins to get boring, then this part will explain how to change the activity to make it more challenging.

Before you sit down for a work session, there are several important points which you should know:

1. Look at the Notes page at the beginning of each section for any instructions. Get any materials you will need ahead of time.
2. A routine is important for the aphasic person. Try to work at the same time and place each day.
3. If you will be using a table, clear off any extra things on it. If there is a design on the table (like a flowered tablecloth), remove it or put something plain like a white towel or pillowcase over it. This way he will be able to see more clearly the things that you put on the table.
4. Turn off the radio or television while you are working. If anyone else is making noise, ask him to go into another room if possible. Even small distractions can make it very hard for the aphasic person to concentrate.

These additional points are important to remember when you are working on the activities:

1. Talk slowly to give the patient time to think about—and understand—what you are saying.
2. You do not need to repeat the directions each time you ask him a question. As soon as he understands what he is supposed to do, then you can stop.
3. Allow him some time to answer a question. It may take the patient longer to think of, or say, what he wants to. Do not interrupt by repeating your question or saying anything until he indicates that he wants help.
4. Encourage him as much as possible. Praise him for what he can do. You do not have to remind him about what he cannot do.
5. If he is having difficulty with an activity, even when it has been simplified, then stop doing it. Do not try to continue, as it will only be frustrating for both of you.

Before you begin a working session then, there are some things to look over ahead of time. The first page of each of the eleven areas will have instructions for you. Your clinician may also have written some notes for you on those pages. You will be working only on those activities which have been checked by your clinician. These may change from time to time as your family member becomes ready for other activities. Be sure to read through the entire activity before you begin. If you do not understand something, ask your speech-language pathologist about it. Do not hesitate to ask questions: your clinician is there to help you.

Understanding

The activities in this section deal with the patient's ability to understand or comprehend what is said to him. Sometimes, even though an aphasic person may seem to understand everything, such is not really the case. This does not mean that his hearing is bad, but it does mean that he does not always understand the information accurately. This section, then, includes activities to help strengthen the ability to make sense out of what the patient hears.

When you talk to the aphasic person, it is important to talk slowly and clearly, but not necessarily loudly. Since these activities are written so that the patient does not have to talk, his answers will be in the form of shaking or nodding the head, pointing, or following a command. However, if the patient is able to speak, then encourage him to answer the questions out loud.

The following kinds of activities are done in this section on Understanding:

Words	Activities 1–7
Descriptions	Activities 8–12
Questions	Activities 13–15, 18, 19
Sentences	Activities 16, 17, 23
Directions	Activities 20–22

Your speech-language pathologist will fill out this part.

Do _____ session(s) each day with the patient.

Do not spend any more than _____ minutes each session working.

_____ Correct any mistakes the patient makes.

_____ Do not correct his mistakes, but continue to the next question.

_____ Repeat the question if he makes a mistake.

_____ Keep track of any errors he makes.

_____ Do not keep track of his errors.

_____ Work on several activities at each working session.

_____ Work on only one activity during each working session.

Notes

_____ **ACTIVITY # 1:** Understanding Words
MATERIALS: none
WHAT TO DO: Name a part of the body. Ask the patient to point to that part of his body.

EXAMPLE:
 If you say "point to your nose"
then he points to his nose.
 If you ask "where is your elbow?
then he points to his elbow.
 Continue by asking about other parts of the body.

_____**ACTIVITY # 2:** Understanding Words
MATERIALS: small objects (see Appendix A)
WHAT TO DO: Place three objects on the table. Name one of them. Ask the patient to point to the one you named.

EXAMPLE:
 Suppose a sock, a ring, and a bar of soap are on the table.
 If you say "point to the ring"
then he does it.

If you ask "which one is the sock?"
then he points to it.

Replace any object he points to with a different one and continue.

SIMPLIFYING THE ACTIVITY: Place two objects on the table instead of three.

EXPANDING THE ACTIVITY: Place four objects on the table instead of three, and continue as before. If his answers remain correct, then add a fifth object. Add more objects until he has difficulty.

—— **ACTIVITY # 3:** Understanding Words

MATERIALS: pictures of objects (see Appendix B)

WHAT TO DO: Place three pictures on the table. Name one of them. Ask the patient to point to the one you named.

EXAMPLE:

Suppose pictures of a pair of skis, a washing machine, and a suitcase are on the table.

If you say "point to the suitcase"
then he does it.

If you ask "which one is the washing machine?"
then he points to the picture of the washer.

Replace any picture he points to with a different one and continue.

SIMPLIFYING THE ACTIVITY: You can place two pictures on the table instead of three. You can also use pictures that are very familiar to the patient.

EXPANDING THE ACTIVITY: Put four pictures on the table instead of three, and continue as before. If his answers remain correct, then add a fifth picture. Add more pictures until he has difficulty.

—— **ACTIVITY # 4:** Understanding Words

MATERIALS: different food items

WHAT TO DO: Place three food items on the table. Name one of them, and ask the patient to point to the item you named.

EXAMPLE:

Suppose a bag of cookies, a box of Wheaties, and a jar of peanut butter are on the table.

If you say "point to the Wheaties"
then he does it.

If you ask "which one is peanut butter?"
then he points to it.

Replace any item he points to with a different one and continue.
VARIATION: You can use coupons with pictures on them instead of actual food products. You can also ask questions about what kind of item it is, such as: vanilla wafers (for cookies), Wheaties (for cereal), and 7-Up (for soft drink).
SIMPLIFYING THE ACTIVITY: Place two food items on the table instead of three.
EXPANDING THE ACTIVITY: Place four food items on the table instead of three, and continue as before. If his answers remain correct, then add a fifth item. Add more items until he has difficulty.

___ ACTIVITY # 5: Understanding Words

MATERIALS: none
WHAT TO DO: Name something in the room that is in full view of the patient. Ask him to point to what you named.

EXAMPLE:
If you say "point to a lamp"
then he does it.
If you ask "where's the TV?"
then he points to it.
Continue by asking other questions.
REMINDER: You may need to suggest that the patient turn his head and look around the room to find what you name.
EXPANDING THE ACTIVITY: Be more specific about what you ask. For instance, you might say "point to the lamp that is on the coffee table" (rather than letting him point to any lamp), or "point to the red ashtray next to the flowers" (rather than letting him point to any ashtray in the room).

___ ACTIVITY # 6: Understanding Words

MATERIALS: action pictures (see Appendix C)
WHAT TO DO: Place a picture on the table. Name something that you see in the picture. Ask the patient to point to what you named.

EXAMPLE:
Suppose the picture shows a man feeding a dog.
If you say "point to the dog's dish"
then he does it.
If you ask "where is the man's belt?"
then he points to it.
Continue with other questions, then change pictures.

_____ **ACTIVITY # 7:** Understanding Words
MATERIALS: a page of advertisements for different products
WHAT TO DO: Place the page of ads on the table. Name one ad, then ask the patient to point to it.

EXAMPLE:
    If you say "show me the ad for shampoo"
    then he points to a shampoo ad on the page.
    If you say "point to the ad for umbrellas"
    then he points to the umbrella ad on the page.
    Continue by asking him to point out other ads. Use another page of ads after you have gone over those on the first page.
VARIATION: If there is more than one ad for a certain product, ask him to find a particular brand name. For instance, if there are two ads for shampoo on the page, you can ask him to point to the ad for either one brand or another.
SIMPLIFYING THE ACTIVITY: You can cut out the ads individually and use only a few at a time. For instance, you might put three ads rather than a whole page on the table. You can fold the page in half to cover some of the ads, or cover them with blank sheets of paper or cardboard.

_____ **ACTIVITY # 8:** Understanding Descriptions
MATERIALS: none
WHAT TO DO: Describe a part of the body. Ask the patient to point to the part you described.

EXAMPLE:
    If you ask "what do you use to smell with?"
    then he points to his nose.
    If you ask "where do you wear a watch?"
    then he points to his wrist.
    Continue by asking about other parts of the body.

_____ **ACTIVITY # 9:** Understanding Descriptions
MATERIALS: small objects (see Appendix A)
WHAT TO DO: Place three objects on the table. Describe how you use one of them. Ask the patient to point to the one that you described.

EXAMPLE:
    Suppose a toothbrush, an eraser, and a sock are on the table. If you say "point to the one you use to clean your teeth"
    then he points to the toothbrush.

If you ask "which one do you wear on your foot?"
then he points to the sock.

Replace any object he points to with a different one and continue.

SIMPLIFYING THE ACTIVITY: Put two objects on the table instead of three.

EXPANDING THE ACTIVITY: Put four objects on the table instead of three, and continue as before. If his answers remain correct, then add a fifth object. Add more objects until he has difficulty.

_____ **ACTIVITY # 10:** Understanding Descriptions
MATERIALS: pictures of objects (see Appendix B)
WHAT TO DO: Place three pictures on the table and describe how you use an item in one of the pictures. Ask the patient to point to the picture that you described.

EXAMPLE:

Suppose pictures of a tractor, a calculator, and a teapot are on the table.

If you say "point to the one a farmer uses in his work"
then he points to the tractor.

If you ask "which one could help you balance a checkbook?"
then he points to the calculator.

Replace any picture he points to with a different one and continue.

SIMPLIFYING THE ACTIVITY: Instead of pictures place two objects on the table (see Appendix A). Continue the activity.

EXPANDING THE ACTIVITY: Put four pictures on the table instead of three, and continue as before. If his answers remain correct, then add a fifth picture. Add more pictures until he has difficulty.

_____ **ACTIVITY # 11:** Understanding Descriptions
MATERIALS: a page of advertisements for different products
WHAT TO DO: Place a page of ads on the table, and describe a product in one of the ads. Ask the patient to point to the product you described.

EXAMPLE:

If you ask "which one is selling something for a car?"
then he points to an ad for tires, a car battery, etc.

If you ask "which ad shows something you wear to keep warm?"
then he points to an ad for gloves, a coat, a hat, or something similar.

Continue asking him to point out other products. Use another page of ads after you have gone over the first page.

SIMPLIFYING THE ACTIVITY: You can cut out the ads individually and use only a few at a time. For instance, place three ads on the table rather than a whole page. You can fold the page in half to cover some of the ads, or cover them with blank sheets of paper or cardboard.

_____ **ACTIVITY # 12:** Understanding Descriptions

MATERIALS: a page of photographs from a newspaper, magazine, or book

WHAT TO DO: Describe one of the pictures to the patient and ask him to point to it.

EXAMPLE:

Suppose the page has photos of several famous entertainers.

If you ask "which picture shows Frank Sinatra singing?"

then he points to it.

If you ask "point to the picture where Burt Reynolds is surrounded by women"

then he points to that one.

Continue with other questions. Use another page of pictures after you have gone over the first page.

SIMPLIFYING THE ACTIVITY: Use only two pictures at one time. Cover the others with white paper or cardboard.

EXPANDING THE ACTIVITY: You can make your descriptions more difficult. For instance, you can identify a picture with a hint, such as a name or a place. You can direct the patient to point to a specific area such as: the one to the left of Frank Sinatra, the third picture from the right, the one that has more than four people in it, etc.

_____ **ACTIVITY # 13:** Understanding Shorter Questions

MATERIALS: none

WHAT TO DO: Ask the patient a short yes-or-no question about himself.

EXAMPLE:

If you ask "are you wearing a red shirt?"

then he answers correctly.

If you ask "are you in a hotel?"

then he answers correctly.

Continue with other questions.

REMINDER: Encourage the patient to answer aloud. If he cannot, ask him to nod or shake his head.

_____ ACTIVITY # 14: Understanding Shorter Questions
MATERIALS: none
WHAT TO DO: Ask the patient a short yes-or-no question. It does not have to be a logical question.

EXAMPLE:
If you ask "does a chair talk?"
then he says no.
If you ask "can you eat raisins?"
then he says yes.
Continue with other questions.
REMINDER: Encourage the patient to answer aloud. If he cannot, ask him to nod or shake his head.

_____ ACTIVITY # 15: Understanding Shorter Questions
MATERIALS: none
WHAT TO DO: Ask the patient a yes-or-no question about a general fact.

EXAMPLE:
If you ask "is Eisenhower now the President?"
then he says no.
If you ask "is Thanksgiving in November?"
then he says yes.
Continue with other questions.
REMINDER: Questions can be about any topic. Encourage the patient to answer aloud. If he cannot, ask him to nod or shake his head.
EXPANDING THE ACTIVITY: You can ask longer questions such as "if you were going to shovel snow, would you use a rake?" You can ask judgment questions such as "is a train heavier than a piano?"

_____ ACTIVITY # 16: Understanding a Sentence
MATERIALS: none
WHAT TO DO: Say a sentence. Some of your sentences need not be logical. Ask the patient to indicate yes if it is true and no if it is not.

EXAMPLE:
If you say "I keep ice cream in the stove"
then he says no.
If you say "a rug goes on the floor"
then he says yes.
If you say "a jewelry store sells hammers"
then he says no.

Continue with other questions.

REMINDER: Encourage the patient to answer aloud. If he cannot, ask him to nod or shake his head.

EXPANDING THE ACTIVITY: Think of sentences which almost sound correct but are not, such as "The Chinese eat a lot of dice" (instead of rice).

_____ **ACTIVITY # 17:** Understanding Sentences

MATERIALS: a dictionary might be helpful

WHAT TO DO: Tell the patient that you will be saying a word and then giving a definition of that word. Ask him to tell you if the definition is correct.

EXAMPLE:

If you say "a stone is a type of meat"
then he says no.
If you say "a star is a bright object in the sky"
then he says yes.
If you say " 'super' is a word meaning great or fantastic"
then he says yes.
Continue with other words and definitions.

REMINDER: You can use the dictionary to find definitions or you can be creative and make up your own definitions.

SIMPLIFYING THE ACTIVITY: Choose familiar words and use definitions which are very different from what the word really means.

_____ **ACTIVITY # 18:** Understanding Questions

MATERIALS: family photographs, preferably ones that include more than just a person's face

WHAT TO DO: Place a photograph on the table. Ask the patient a yes-or-no question about the photo.

EXAMPLE:

If you ask "was it taken in winter?"
then he answers correctly.
If you ask "does it show two people waving?"
then he answers correctly.
If you ask "is Aunt Mary in the picture?"
then he answers correctly.
Ask other questions about the same photo, then change photos and continue as before.

REMINDER: Encourage the patient to answer aloud. If he cannot, ask him to nod or shake his head.

ACTIVITY # 19: Understanding Questions

MATERIALS: family photographs, preferably ones that include more than just a person's face

WHAT TO DO: Place three photos on the table. Ask the patient a question that he can answer by pointing to one of the photos.

EXAMPLE:

If you ask "which one was taken at your birthday party?"
then he points to the correct photo.

If you say "point to the one taken in Chicago"
then he points to the correct one.

Replace any photo he points to with a different one and continue.

SIMPLIFYING THE ACTIVITY: Place two photos on the table instead of three.

EXPANDING THE ACTIVITY: Place four photos on the table instead of three, and continue as before. If the patient's answers remain correct, then add a fifth photo. Add more photos until he has difficulty.

ACTIVITY # 20: Understanding Shorter Directions

MATERIALS: none

WHAT TO DO: Tell the patient that you are going to ask him to do what you say.

EXAMPLE:

If you say "blink your eyes"
then he does it.

If you say "make a fist"
then he does it.

Continue with other directions.

ACTIVITY # 21: Understanding Directions

MATERIALS: small objects (see Appendix A)

WHAT TO DO: Place three objects on the table. Ask the patient to move one or more of the objects.

EXAMPLE:

Suppose a glass, a nickel, and a pencil are on the table.

If you say "put the pen in the glass"
then he does it.

If you say "turn over the nickel"
then he turns it over.

If you say "give me the pencil"
then he does it.

Continue with more directions, then change objects.

SIMPLIFYING THE ACTIVITY: Place two objects on the table instead of three.

EXPANDING THE ACTIVITY: Place four objects on the table instead of three, and continue as before. If his answers remain correct, then add a fifth object. Add more objects until he has difficulty.

_____ **ACTIVITY # 22:** Understanding Directions

MATERIALS: pencil and unlined paper

WHAT TO DO: Put the pencil and paper in front of the patient, and ask him to follow your directions.

EXAMPLE:

If you say "make a small circle in the center of the paper"
then he does it.

If you say "put two checks under the circle"
then he does it.

If you say "put a 5 in the bottom left corner of the paper"
then he does it.

Continue with other directions.

REMINDER: You can give the patient many directions to follow.

VARIATION: If the patient can spell, then ask him to write words. If he cannot, then ask him to draw squares, circles, triangles, lines, and numbers.

EXPANDING THE ACTIVITY: You can make the directions longer, such as "make three lines in the top half of the page and make the line in the middle the shortest and the other two longer." You can make the directions involve some thinking, such as "if flies are larger than elephants, then draw a small circle in one of the corners of the page. If they are not, then draw a small square in the center of the page."

_____ **ACTIVITY # 23:** Understanding Sentences

MATERIALS: none, although you can use sentences from books or magazines

WHAT TO DO: Tell the patient to listen while you say one or two sentences. Pause, then ask him yes-or-no questions about what you said. Ask questions that he can answer by shaking or nodding his head.

EXAMPLE:

Suppose your sentence is "the paperboy delivered the paper at seven-thirty this morning."

If you ask "did the paperboy come at eight-thirty?" *then he answers no.*

If you ask "did he bring the paper?" *then he answers no.*

Suppose your sentence is "Acadia National Park is located in Maine and covers over 41,000 acres of land."

If you ask "is Acadia National Park in Vermont?" *then he answers no.*

If you ask "does this park have over 41,000 acres of land?" *then he answers yes.*

Continue with other sentences.

REMINDER: Sentences that give any kind of information may be used. Encourage the patient to answer aloud. If he cannot, ask him to nod or shake his head.

SIMPLIFYING THE ACTIVITY: Use one short sentence such as "the cougar is a wild animal." Ask questions such as "is the cougar a tame animal?" or "am I talking about a tiger?"

Other Activities

Repeating

Sometimes an aphasic person may not be able to begin a word (or conversation) but may be able to repeat sentences. At other times he may be able to talk quite well but may have trouble repeating short phrases. The activities in this section will concentrate on the patient's ability to imitate or repeat exactly what is said.

Being able to repeat can be a step toward being able to initiate speech. It is helpful to realize that the aphasic person's ability to imitate may be very inconsistent. He may be able to do an activity very well at one time and then find it hard to do the same activity at another time. The activities in this section range in difficulty from imitating a movement to repeating long directions.

The following kinds of activities are done in this section on Repeating:

Imitating Movements	Activities 24–26
Sounds	Activity 27
Syllables	Activities 28–29
Singing	Activity 30
Reciting	Activity 31
Words	Activities 32–34
Numbers	Activities 35–37
Phrases	Activities 38–40
Sentences	Activities 41–48
Pausing and Repeating	Activity 49

Your speech-language pathologist will fill out this part.

Do _____ session(s) each day with the patient.

Do not spend any more than _____ minutes each session working.

_____ Correct any mistakes he makes.

_____ Do not correct his mistakes, but continue to the next question.

_____ Repeat the question if he makes a mistake.

_____ Keep track of any errors he makes.

_____ Do not keep track of his errors.

_____ Work on several activities at each working session.

_____ Work on only one activity during each working session.

Notes

_____ **ACTIVITY # 24:** Imitating Movements

MATERIALS: none

WHAT TO DO: Your clinician has checked some movements to practice. Choose one and tell the patient to watch you do the movement.
Then ask him to imitate what you just did.

EXAMPLE:

_____ Put up different numbers of fingers.

_____ Point to parts of the body.

_____ Make some common gestures.

_____ Clap your hands or slap your knee several times.

_____ Clap your hands or slap your knee in a certain rhythm.

REMINDER: Encourage the patient to watch closely while you show him what to do.
VARIATION: Work on only one of the movements or work on several during one session.
SIMPLIFYING THE ACTIVITY: Do the movements along with the patient.

_____ **ACTIVITY # 25:** Imitating Movements
MATERIALS: none
WHAT TO DO: Your clinician has checked some movements to practice. Choose one and tell the patient to watch you do the movement. Then ask him to imitate what you just did.

EXAMPLE:
_____ Open your mouth very wide.
_____ Press your lips together.
_____ Smile.
_____ Open, then close your mouth.
_____ Stick out your tongue.
_____ Clench your teeth.
_____ Put your tongue between your teeth.
_____ Pucker your lips.
_____ Lick your lips.
_____ Puff up your cheeks.
_____ Clear your throat.
_____ Sigh.
_____ Cough.
_____ Hum a tune.
REMINDER: Encourage the patient to watch closely while you show him what to do.
VARIATION: Work on only one movement, or work on several during one session.
SIMPLIFYING THE ACTIVITY: Do the movements along with the patient.
EXPANDING THE ACTIVITY: Do the movements as fast as the patient can imitate you. Alternate different movements and have him imitate one after another.

_____ **ACTIVITY # 26:** Imitating Movements
MATERIALS: none
WHAT TO DO: Pretend you are doing something, but do not use any props. Tell the patient to watch, then ask him to imitate what you just did.

EXAMPLE:

If you pretend you are combing your hair
then he does the same thing.

If you pantomime brushing your teeth
then he does the same thing.

If you act as if you are catching a ball
then he does the same thing.

Continue to pantomime other actions.

REMINDER: You will not be using any materials with this activity, but just pretending to do some kind of action. Encourage the patient to watch closely while you pantomime.

SIMPLIFYING THE ACTIVITY: Use simple actions such as crossing your arms, touching your forehead, etc.

EXPANDING THE ACTIVITY: Use actions that take a few steps to imitate, such as breaking and scrambling an egg, wrapping a gift, etc.

_____ **ACTIVITY # 27:** Repeating Sounds

MATERIALS: none

WHAT TO DO: Tell the patient to watch and listen. Make a sound and hold it for about five seconds, then ask him to make the same sound and hold the sound as long as he can.

EXAMPLE:

Some sounds include: ah, oh, ee (as in bee), mmm, ssss, sshh (as in she), oo (as in moon), zzz (as in zoo), uh, nnn.

REMINDER: Some of the sounds will probably be easier for the patient to make than others. Your clinician may ask you to try all of the sounds, concentrate on certain ones, or add others.

VARIATION: Time the patient on how long he is able to hold a sound. The next time, have him hold it longer.

_____ **ACTIVITY # 28:** Repeating Syllables

MATERIALS: none, but your clinician may give you a list to use

WHAT TO DO: Say a syllable while the patient watches and listens. Ask him to repeat what you said.

EXAMPLE:

Some syllables include: can, day, oh, ha, go, be, to, mom, bow, lie, knee.

REMINDER: If the patient says the word incorrectly, then repeat the word slowly and ask him to try it again.

SIMPLIFYING THE ACTIVITY: Say the syllable or word, then say the word with him. Repeat it along with him. Fade out your voice if he can finish the word on his own.

EXPANDING THE ACTIVITY: You can say the words as quickly as he can imitate the sound. You can also use many different words and have him imitate one after another.

_____ **ACTIVITY # 29:** Repeating Syllables
MATERIALS: none, but your clinician may give you a list to use
WHAT TO DO: Say a syllable three times in a row, then ask the patient to repeat what you just said.

EXAMPLE:
   Some syllables include: be, ha, toe, ma, low, la, so, the, ray, pen, mow, ox.
VARIATION: Say three different syllables which are to be repeated, such as: toe, be, la.
EXPANDING THE ACTIVITY: Say the syllables five times in a row quickly. Ask the patient to repeat them as fast as he can.

_____ **ACTIVITY # 30:** Singing
MATERIALS: none
WHAT TO DO: Pick a song that the patient knows. Begin by singing the first bar or two. Ask him to sing with you, then start again very slowly. He may not be able to sing each word but let him fade in and out wherever he can.

EXAMPLE:
   Some songs include: "America"; "Bicycle Built for Two"; "For He's a Jolly Good Fellow"; "Happy Birthday"; "Home on the Range"; "I've Been Working on the Railroad"; "Let Me Call You Sweetheart"; various Christmas carols; hymns; songs from musicals; other familiar songs.
REMINDER: These songs are only examples. Your clinician may add some or you may think of others. You may find that the patient can sing some songs very well but has trouble with others. Try several to see which ones are easier.
SIMPLIFYING THE ACTIVITY: If the patient cannot sing any words, encourage him to follow the tune or rhythm. You can hold his hand and tap out the rhythm for him as you sing.
EXPANDING THE ACTIVITY: Tell the patient what song to sing, and let him sing it by himself. You can help him start the song if necessary.

_____ **ACTIVITY # 31:** Reciting
MATERIALS: none
WHAT TO DO: Your clinician has checked some examples for you to recite. Tell the patient what you are going to recite, and begin slowly. Encourage him to say it with you. Start out together, but fade out your voice when you can.

EXAMPLE:
_____ Counting
_____ Alphabet
_____ Days of the week
_____ Months of the year
_____ Pledge of Allegiance
_____ Short rhymes (like nursery rhymes or limericks)
_____ Lord's Prayer (or other familiar prayers)
_____ Any poem, speech, creed, or rules that the patient has learned
_____ Famous quotes
_____ Commercial jingles or ads
_____ Bible verses

REMINDER: Recite slowly, and encourage the patient to watch you. If he can say it on his own, then fade out your voice but keep mouthing the words. If he gets stuck, then recite aloud along with him until you feel you can fade out your voice again.
SIMPLIFYING THE ACTIVITY: Do not try to fade out your voice. Recite slowly and clearly while the patient recites with you.
EXPANDING THE ACTIVITY: Help the patient with the first few words, then stop and let him continue on his own. Do not mouth the words, but let him say them by himself. If he gets stuck, help him at that point or have him start over again.

_____ **ACTIVITY # 32:** Repeating Words
MATERIALS: none, but your clinician may give you a list to use
WHAT TO DO: Your clinician has checked some of the following examples to practice. Say a word while the patient watches and listens, then ask him to repeat it.

EXAMPLE:
_____ Word list from your clinician
_____ Letters
_____ Numbers
_____ One-syllable words
_____ Words beginning with a certain sound
_____ Common everyday words
_____ Names of persons or places

_____ Hard to pronounce words
_____ Words from indexes, puzzles, etc.
REMINDER: If the patient does not say the word correctly, then repeat the word slowly and have him try it again.
SIMPLIFYING THE ACTIVITY: First say the word for the patient, then say it with him. Repeat it again along with him. If you can fade out your voice so that he finishes the word on his own, then do so.

_____ **ACTIVITY # 33:** Repeating Longer Words
MATERIALS: a dictionary
WHAT TO DO: Use the dictionary to find either long or hard-to-pronounce words. Say a word slowly so that the patient is able to hear each syllable, then ask him to repeat it.

EXAMPLE:
    If you say "linoleum" slowly
then he says it.
    If you say "metropolitan" slowly
then he says it.
    Continue with other words.
REMINDER: If the patient has trouble saying the word, repeat it again slowly for him.
SIMPLIFYING THE ACTIVITY: Say one syllable at a time, and let the patient repeat each syllable. If he can do that, try two syllables at a time. Work this way until he says the entire word. If he cannot say two syllables together, then stop and go on to another word.
EXPANDING THE ACTIVITY: Say the word at normal speed without emphasizing any sounds or syllables.

_____ **ACTIVITY # 34:** Repeating Words
MATERIALS: none
WHAT TO DO: Ask the patient a question that includes a choice of a right and wrong answer. Ask him to answer correctly.

EXAMPLE:
    If you ask "is Thanksgiving in November or January?"
then he says "November."
    If you ask "do you read or eat a book?"
then he says "read."
    If you ask "do you listen to a curtain or to a radio?"
then he says "radio."
    Continue with other questions.

_____ ACTIVITY # 35: Repeating Numbers
MATERIALS: none
WHAT TO DO: Say two different numbers, one after the other. Ask the patient to repeat what you said. Use numbers from zero to nine.

EXAMPLE:
  If you say "two, nine"
then he says "two, nine."
  Continue with other combinations of numbers under ten.
EXPANDING THE ACTIVITY: You can say three numbers instead of two. You can say two numbers that are between ten and one hundred.

_____ ACTIVITY # 36: Repeating Numbers
MATERIALS: none
WHAT TO DO: Say four different numbers, one after the other. Ask the patient to repeat what you said. Use numbers from zero to nine.

EXAMPLE:
  If you say "six, two, seven, nine"
then he says "six, two, seven, nine."
  Continue with other combinations of numbers under ten.
SIMPLIFYING THE ACTIVITY: Say the numbers in small groups for the patient to repeat. For instance, you can say "six, two," then "seven, nine."
EXPANDING THE ACTIVITY: Your clinician may have checked the following examples to practice.
  _____ Five numbers in a row (as in zip codes)
  _____ Six numbers in a row (as on some license plates and in combination with letters)
  _____ Seven numbers in a row (as in telephone numbers)
  _____ Numbers between ten and one hundred

_____ ACTIVITY # 37: Repeating Numbers
MATERIALS: none
WHAT TO DO: Say an amount of money, and ask the patient to repeat what you said. Start with smaller amounts and work up to larger ones.

EXAMPLE:
  If you say "fourteen cents"
then he says it.

If you say "seventy-nine dollars and thirty-three cents"
then he says it.
Continue by saying other amounts of money.

_____ **ACTIVITY # 38:** Repeating Phrases
MATERIALS: none
WHAT TO DO: Your clinician has checked some facts to practice.
Say one of the facts to the patient, then ask him to repeat what you
said.

EXAMPLE:
_____ Patient's name
_____ The day, month, and year
_____ His address
_____ His phone number
_____ Names of other family members
_____ Names of relatives and/or friends
_____ Words describing the weather
_____ Cities or streets in the area
_____ His place of employment
_____ His bank, insurance company, etc.
_____ Professional people he sees (doctors, dentists, etc.)
_____ Organizations to which he belongs
SIMPLIFYING THE ACTIVITY: Break the information into parts
so that the patient can repeat a little bit at a time. If he is able to say
each part separately, then ask him to repeat a little more. If he can't,
then continue to repeat the facts a few at a time.

_____ **ACTIVITY # 39:** Repeating Phrases
MATERIALS: none
WHAT TO DO: Say a short phrase, then ask the patient to repeat
what you said.

EXAMPLE:
If you say "a red sock"
then he says it.
If you say "a cup of soup"
then he says it.
Continue with other phrases.
VARIATION: If the patient has a particular area of interest, then
you can use phrases related to it. Some areas of interest include: cooking, cars, sewing, computers, business, medicine, sports, woodworking,
antiques.

_____ **ACTIVITY # 40:** Repeating Phrases

MATERIALS: see checked examples

WHAT TO DO: Your clinician has checked some items for you to use. Choose a phrase and say it out loud. Ask the patient to repeat exactly what you said.

EXAMPLE:

_____ Addresses

_____ Want ads in a newspaper

_____ Descriptions of homes or apartments for sale

_____ Definitions from crossword puzzles

_____ Titles of news or magazine articles

_____ Book or song titles

_____ Names of famous people

_____ TV programs (the title, stars, time, and channel)

_____ Ingredients listed on a package or bottle

_____ Recipe names and ingredients

REMINDER: You may find it is easier for the patient to repeat some things than to repeat others, even though they might be the same length.

SIMPLIFYING THE ACTIVITY: Have the patient repeat things that are short. For instance, ask him to repeat one ingredient listed in spaghetti sauce rather than three at a time.

EXPANDING THE ACTIVITY: Have him repeat entire descriptions instead of phrases. For instance, read an entire want ad, then ask him to repeat it.

_____ **ACTIVITY # 41:** Repeating Sentences

MATERIALS: none

WHAT TO DO: This activity is to be done whenever it seems appropriate. There will be times during the day when you and the patient will be doing things together, and then you can practice this exercise. Say a sentence that describes something the patient is going to do or is already doing. Ask him to repeat what you said.

EXAMPLE:

If the patient is drinking a glass of water, you can say "I am drinking a glass of water"
then he repeats it.

If he is going to look at TV, you can say "I'm going to watch TV"
then he repeats it.

Continue with other sentences throughout the day for him to repeat.

REMINDER: Do not ask the patient to repeat everything he is doing.

Do not ask him to repeat a sentence if he is concentrating on something else. This activity should be done before the patient starts, when he takes a break from, or when he finishes his task.

SIMPLIFYING THE ACTIVITY: Use a phrase or a word instead of a sentence to describe what the patient is doing.

_____ **ACTIVITY # 42:** Repeating Sentences

MATERIALS: none

WHAT TO DO: Say a short sentence, and ask the patient to repeat what you said.

EXAMPLE:

If you say "today is Tuesday"
then he repeats it.
If you say "we are out of milk"
then he repeats it.
Continue with other sentences.

REMINDER: Try not to make your sentences longer than eight words.

_____ **ACTIVITY # 43:** Repeating Longer Sentences

MATERIALS: none

WHAT TO DO: Say a short sentence about anything, then ask the patient to repeat it. Now say the sentence again but add some new information. Then ask him to repeat the new sentence.

EXAMPLE:

If you say "I like popcorn"
then he repeats it.
If you then say "I like popcorn and butter"
he repeats that.
If you say "the green car has a dent"
then he repeats it.
If you then say "the green car has a dent on the left front fender"
he repeats that.
Continue with other sentences.

REMINDER: Always repeat the original sentence you say along with the new information.

EXPANDING THE ACTIVITY: Add more information to the original sentence. For instance, you can add to the first sentence as follows: "I like salted popcorn and butter"; "when I go to the movies I like salted popcorn and butter"; "when I go to the movies I like to buy something to drink with my salted popcorn and butter." When the sentence becomes too long for him to repeat, then stop and start with a new, short sentence.

_____ **ACTIVITY # 44:** Repeating Longer Sentences
MATERIALS: action pictures (see Appendix C)
WHAT TO DO: Place a picture on the table. Say a sentence that describes something in the picture, and then ask the patient to repeat what you said.

EXAMPLE:
Suppose the picture includes a family having a picnic.
If you point to a part of the picture and say "the child is eating a hot dog"
then he repeats it.
If you say "the picture was taken on a warm day"
then he repeats it.
Continue with other sentences, then change the picture.

_____ **ACTIVITY # 45:** Repeating Longer Sentences
MATERIALS: none, but you can use a book, magazine, or newspaper to get ideas for sentences to use
WHAT TO DO: Say a sentence of average length about anything you want. Ask the patient to repeat what you said.

EXAMPLE:
If you say "the humidifier in the furnace isn't working"
then he repeats it.
If you say "the President's speech was twenty minutes long"
then he repeats your sentence.
Continue with other sentences.
SIMPLIFYING THE ACTIVITY: You can use sentences which are shorter. You can break down your sentence into parts and have the patient repeat them one at a time.
EXPANDING THE ACTIVITY: You can use sentences which are longer or use more difficult vocabulary, numbers or dates, or sentences taken directly from an article.

_____ **ACTIVITY # 46:** Repeating Longer Sentences
MATERIALS: see checked examples
WHAT TO DO: Your clinician has checked some examples to practice. Read a sentence out loud, then ask the patient to repeat it exactly as you read it.

EXAMPLE:

_____ Instructions on a product

_____ Recipe directions

_____ Definitions from a dictionary

_____ Horoscopes

_____ Descriptions of items in a catalog

_____ Photograph or cartoon captions

_____ **ACTIVITY # 47:** Repeating Tongue Twisters

MATERIALS: none, but your clinician may give you a list to use

WHAT TO DO: Say a tongue twister, and ask the patient to repeat what you said. (Probably the most popular tongue twister is "Peter Piper picked a peck of pickled peppers.")

EXAMPLE:

If you say "Tom tasted two turnips"
then he repeats it.

If you say "Sam Smith saw Sue on Sunday"
then he repeats it.

Continue with other tongue twisters.

REMINDER: You can use the dictionary to help think of words that begin with the same letter. The sentences do not really have to make much sense, as long as they are hard to say.

EXPANDING THE ACTIVITY: You can ask him to repeat the tongue twister two times in a row. You can ask him to say it as fast as he can.

_____ **ACTIVITY # 48:** Repeating Longer Sentences

MATERIALS: none

WHAT TO DO: Say a sentence that gives some directions and ask the patient to repeat it.

EXAMPLE:

If you say "go two blocks and turn right at the traffic light"
then he repeats it.

If you say "if you can't reach me in my office by five o'clock, call me at home after seven-thirty"
then he repeats it.

Continue with other directions.

SIMPLIFYING THE ACTIVITY: You can use directions which are familiar to the patient. You can make the directions shorter and simpler with few numbers in them.

EXPANDING THE ACTIVITY: You can say directions which are

unfamiliar. You can use any numbers, amounts, dates, etc. You can also use the kind of direction you might get from someone if you were lost.

_____ **ACTIVITY # 49:** Pausing and Repeating
MATERIALS: none
WHAT TO DO: This activity can be used with any other in this section. Follow the directions for the other activity, but make the patient pause before he repeats what you said. You are going to ask him to repeat what you say, but before he begins to repeat, put your hand in front of his face for a few seconds and tell him not to speak until you put your hand down. Then have him repeat what he heard.

EXAMPLE:

Suppose you are asking him to repeat the syllable oh.

You say "oh" and quickly put your hand in front of his face. After two or three seconds, you put your hand down
then he repeats oh.

Suppose you are asking him to repeat the sentence "the mailman was early today."

You say the sentence, put up your hand, and wait two or three seconds. When your hand goes down
then he says "the mailman was early today."

Other Activities

Nonverbal Communication

This section deals with different forms of nonverbal communication, getting a message across without talking. We can communicate nonverbally with body language, facial expressions, gestures, pointing, drawing, pantomiming, etc.

If the aphasic person is not able to communicate well by talking, then the activities in this part may be helpful in developing other means of conveying information. Your clinician will check any which should be tried.

The following kinds of activities are done in this section on Nonverbal Communication:

Expressing Yes and No	Activities 50–52
Pointing	Activities 53–54
Imitating	Activities 55–56
Using a Nonverbal Communication Aid	Activity 58
Pantomiming	Activities 57,59–61
Drawing	Activities 62–63
Conveying Information	Activities 64–66

Your speech-language pathologist will fill out this part.

Do _____ session(s) each day with the patient.

Do not spend any more than _____ minutes each session working.

_____ Correct any mistakes he makes.

_____ Do not correct his mistakes, but continue to the next question.

_____ Repeat the question if he makes a mistake.

_____ Keep track of any errors he makes.

_____ Do not keep track of his errors.

_____ Work on several activities at each working session.

_____ Work on only one activity during each working session.

Notes

_____ **ACTIVITY # 50:** Nodding Yes

MATERIALS: none

WHAT TO DO: Say yes while you are nodding your head, then ask the patient to nod his head yes. If he does not, move his head up and down with your hands while you say yes. Practice this until he nods his head when you say yes.

_____ **ACTIVITY # 51:** Shaking No
MATERIALS: none
WHAT TO DO: Say no while you are shaking your head, then ask him to shake his head no. If he does not, move his head from side to side with your hands while you say no. Practice this until he shakes his head when you say no.

_____ **ACTIVITY # 52:** Expressing Yes and No
MATERIALS: none
WHAT TO DO: Practice nodding yes and shaking no.

EXAMPLE:
   If you say "tell me no"
then he nods his head no.
   If you say "tell me yes"
then he shakes his head yes.
   Continue practicing this until the patient is able to respond to yes or no on command.

_____ **ACTIVITY # 53:** Pointing
MATERIALS: none
WHAT TO DO: Tell the patient to point to his nose while you take his hand and move it to his nose. Do this a few times, saying "point to your nose" as you move his hand to his nose. Next, make sure his hand is down and say "point to your nose." If he points correctly, make sure his hand is down, then ask him again. If he does not point correctly, take his hand and repeat from the beginning. If he does point correctly, continue to practice until he responds on command.

_____ **ACTIVITY # 54:** Pointing
MATERIALS: a small object
WHAT TO DO: Place an object, such as a book, on the table. Tell him to point to the book while you take his hand and move it to the book. Do this a few times, saying "point to the book" as you move his hand to the book. Next, make sure his hand is down and say "point to the book." If he points correctly, make sure his hand is down, then ask him again. If he does not point correctly, take his hand and re-peat from the beginning. If he does point correctly, continue to prac-tice until he responds on command.

_____**ACTIVITY # 55:** Imitating a Gesture
MATERIALS: none
WHAT TO DO: Ask the patient to watch while you make a gesture, then ask him to imitate what you did.

EXAMPLE:
If you wave your hand
then he waves his hand.
If you cross your arms
then he crosses his arms.
Continue with other gestures.
REMINDER: Use any kind of gesture for the patient to imitate.

_____ **ACTIVITY # 56:** Imitating the Use of an Object
MATERIALS: small objects (see Appendix A)
WHAT TO DO: Pick up one of the objects and demonstrate its use. Then give the object to the patient and ask him to imitate what you did.

EXAMPLE:
Suppose you use a book. You open the book and pretend you are reading it by allowing your head to follow your gaze down the page, and then turning the page. Give the book to the patient
who then imitates how a book is used.
Suppose you are using a tissue. Pick up the tissue and pretend that you are blowing your nose. Give a tissue to the patient
who then imitates what you did.
Continue with other objects.

_____ **ACTIVITY # 57:** Pantomiming
MATERIALS: small objects (see Appendix A)
WHAT TO DO: Give the patient an object, and ask him to show you how to use it.

EXAMPLE:
If you give him a spoon
then he pretends he is eating with it.
If you give him a pencil
then he pretends he is writing with it.
Continue by giving him other objects to demonstrate.
REMINDER: The patient is to demonstrate how to use the object without talking.

_____ **ACTIVITY # 58:** Using a Nonverbal Communication Aid
MATERIALS: a nonverbal communication aid
WHAT TO DO: Follow the instructions of your clinician (see the Notes page).

_____ **ACTIVITY # 59:** Recognizing Pantomime
MATERIALS: pictures of objects (see Appendix B)
WHAT TO DO: Place three pictures on the table. Pretend you are using one of the objects shown in the pictures but do not indicate which one. Ask the patient to point to the appropriate picture.

EXAMPLE:
   Suppose pictures of a lawnmower, a frying pan, and a mirror are on the table.
   If you stand up, pretend you are pushing something, turn around, and push something back
then he points to the picture of the lawnmower.
   If you hold one hand up in front of you, look toward that hand, and pat your hair with the other hand
then he points to the picture of the mirror.
   Replace any picture he points to with a different one and continue.

_____ **ACTIVITY # 60:** Pantomiming
MATERIALS: pictures of objects (see Appendix B)
WHAT TO DO: Place a picture on the table. Ask the patient to show you how to use what is shown.

EXAMPLE:
   If a picture of a broom is on the table
then he pretends he is holding a broom and is sweeping the floor with it.
   If a picture of a sponge is on the table
then he acts as if he is holding a sponge in his hand and cleaning something with it.
   Continue with other pictures for him to pantomime.
REMINDER: The patient is to demonstrate how to use the object without talking.

_____ **ACTIVITY # 61:** Pantomiming
MATERIALS: none
WHAT TO DO: Name an object, then ask the patient to show you how he would use that object.

EXAMPLE:

If you say "show me how you use a cup"
then he pretends he is holding a cup in his hands and brings it to his mouth as if he is drinking from it.

If you say "show me how you use a screwdriver"
then he acts as if he is holding one and using it.

Continue by asking him to demonstrate the use of other objects.
REMINDER: The patient is to demonstrate how to use the object without talking.

_____ **ACTIVITY # 62:** Drawing a Small Object
MATERIALS: pencil and paper, small objects (see Appendix A)
WHAT TO DO: Place an object on the table, and ask the patient to draw it. Tell him his drawing does not need to be perfect, only recognizable. When he is finished, put another object on the table for him to draw.
SIMPLIFYING THE ACTIVITY: Begin with objects that are easy to draw, such as a glass, ball, candle, etc.
EXPANDING THE ACTIVITY: Once you can recognize the objects, use things that are a little more difficult to draw, such as a shoe, a watch, or a pair of scissors.

_____ **ACTIVITY # 63:** Drawing a More Complex Object
MATERIALS: paper and pencil, pictures of objects (see Appendix B)
WHAT TO DO: Give the patient the pictures, and ask him to choose something to draw. Tell him not to show you what he has chosen. When he has finished drawing the picture, then you guess what it is. He may need to add more lines to the drawing or give you a hint if you have trouble guessing.

Continue by asking him to draw another one of the pictures.
REMINDER: Tell him that his drawing does not need to be perfect, only recognizable.
SIMPLIFYING THE ACTIVITY: Give him five pictures that are not too hard to draw. Ask him to choose one of the pictures and draw it.
EXPANDING THE ACTIVITY: Do not use pictures. Ask the patient to draw any object. When he has finished, then you guess what it is.

_____ **ACTIVITY # 64:** Conveying Information
MATERIALS: paper and pencil
WHAT TO DO: Ask the patient to show you how he would convey a message. Give him a situation and encourage him to answer in any way that he can. He can gesture, write, point, draw, pantomime, talk, or do anything else.

EXAMPLE:

If you ask "how would you let me know that you are hungry?" *then he might do one of several things—he can point to his mouth, pretend he is eating, say "food" or "hungry," point to some food that he can see, go to the kitchen and open the refrigerator, or draw a picture of some kind of food.*

If you ask "how would you let me know if you have a headache?" *then he might do one of several things—he can put his hand to his head, pound his forehead with his fist, groan and hold his head, say "headache," or get some aspirin.*

Continue by asking him about other situations.

REMINDER: If the patient has trouble answering, encourage him to use other methods of communicating besides talking. There are probably lots of messages that he wants to convey to you during a day: use these as situations for this activity.

_____ **ACTIVITY # 65:** Conveying Information

MATERIALS: pictures of objects (see Appendix B)

WHAT TO DO: Give the pictures to the patient and tell him to turn them over or put them where you cannot see them. He is to look at the first picture and convey to you in some way what the picture shows. You should be able to tell what the picture is, based on the information he gives you.

EXAMPLE:

If the patient has a picture of a rabbit

then he tries to make it clear that you will say "you have a picture of a rabbit." He can do any of several things to get the message across to you. He might get up and hop and twitch his nose. He might say "Easter" or "bunny." He might try to write the word, or he might point to his "hair" (hare).

Continue by having him choose another picture.

REMINDER: If you do not have any idea what he is trying to get across, then you can ask him a question, which he can answer with a yes or a no. Encourage him to use other methods of communication besides talking.

_____ **ACTIVITY # 66:** Conveying Information

MATERIALS: Your clinician may be working on specific gestures, clues, or signals with the patient. This activity is included to help you practice these signals with him. Read the directions on the Notes page.

VARIATION: You can think of your own signals or gestures. For instance, if the patient drools, you can signal to him that he needs to wipe his mouth by touching the corner of your own mouth.

Other Activities

Naming

Just as we sometimes forget a person's name, or a restaurant, so does the aphasic patient—only more so. Someone with aphasia may find it hard to recall the words for persons, places, or things. This section has activities for this kind of difficulty.

These activities can be answered in a single word but provide practice for eventually talking in sentences.

The following kinds of activities are done in this section on Naming:

Completing Phrases/Sentences	Activities 67–68
Word Association	Activities 69–71, 73–77
Identifying Objects/Facts	Activities 72, 78–80
Naming an Item	Activities 81–83

Your speech-language pathologist will fill out this part.

Do _____ session(s) each day with the patient.

Do not spend any more than _____ minutes each session working.

_____ Correct any mistakes, but continue to the next question.

_____ Do not correct his mistakes, but continue to the next question.

_____ Repeat the question if he makes a mistake.

_____ Keep track of any errors he makes.

_____ Do not keep track of his errors.

_____ Work on several activities at each working session.

_____ Work on only one activity during each working session.

Notes

_____ **ACTIVITY # 67:** Completing a Phrase
MATERIALS: none
WHAT TO DO: Say the first half of a familiar phrase, pause, and wait for the patient to finish the phrase with a word that makes sense.

EXAMPLE:
    If you say "comb and . . ."
then he says "brush."
    If you say "Romeo and . . ."
then he says "Juliet."
    Continue with other phrases.

_____ **ACTIVITY # 68:** Completing a Sentence
MATERIALS: none
WHAT TO DO: The patient is to complete your sentence with one or more words. You say the beginning of a sentence, then the patient is to supply the last word(s) of the sentence so that it makes sense.

EXAMPLE:
    If you say "you can read a . . ."
then he can say "book," "magazine," "novel," "letter," "sign," or another word that makes sense.
    If you say "the ship was lost during the . . ."
then he can say "terrible storm," "hurricane," "war," or another word that makes sense.
    Continue with other sentences.
REMINDER: If you have trouble thinking of sentences, use a book or magazine.
SIMPLIFYING THE ACTIVITY: Use sentences in which only one or two words will make sense, such as "the color of the American flag is red, white and . . ."

_____ **ACTIVITY # 69:** Associating Objects and Words
MATERIALS: none
WHAT TO DO: Say the name of an object, then ask the patient to name things that are a part of that object.

EXAMPLE:
    If you say "book"
then he can say "page," "cover," "words," "paper," or other parts of a book.
    If you say "rose bush"
then he can say "petals," "leaves," "stems," "thorns," "roots," or other parts of a rose bush.
    Continue by naming other objects.

VARIATION: Use pictures of objects (see Appendix B).
SIMPLIFYING THE ACTIVITY: Use pictures of objects (see Appendix B). Point to different parts of the object and ask him to name them.

_____ **ACTIVITY # 70:** Associating Words
MATERIALS: none
WHAT TO DO: Say a word. Ask the patient to say any words that can describe your word.

EXAMPLE:
 If you say "golf ball"
then he can say "small," "round," "hard," "white," or other words that describe it.
 If you say "pillow"
then he can say "soft," "foam," "feathers," "case," or other words that describe it.
 Continue with other words.

_____ **ACTIVITY # 71:** Associating Words
MATERIALS: none
WHAT TO DO: Say a word. Ask the patient to say other words that come to his mind.

EXAMPLE:
 If you say "drive"
then he can say "car," "shaft," "bus," "chauffeur," "golf," "trip," "driveway," "circular," or other words related to drive.
 If you say "award"
then he can say "Academy," "first prize," "trophy," "banquet," or other words related to award.
 Continue with other words.

_____ **ACTIVITY # 72:** Identifying Objects
MATERIALS: see checked examples
WHAT TO DO: Your clinician has checked some examples to practice. Point to something and ask the patient to name what you have shown him.

EXAMPLE:
 _____ Pictures of objects (see Appendix B)
 _____ Small objects (see Appendix A)

_____ Objects in your room
_____ Objects in any part of the house or hospital
_____ Parts of the body
_____ Foods
_____ Photographs of relatives or friends
_____ Photographs of famous people (in magazines or papers)
_____ Action pictures (see Appendix C)

_____ **ACTIVITY # 73:** Associating Words
MATERIALS: none
WHAT TO DO: Think of a category and ask the patient to name something in that category.

EXAMPLE:
     If you say "fruits"
then he names any fruit.
     If you say "appliances"
then he names any appliance.
     Continue by naming other categories.
REMINDER: Choose a category which is broad (such as foods), specific (such as kinds of candy bars), or narrow (such as a president since 1970).
EXPANDING THE ACTIVITY: Ask the patient to name two or more things in each category.

_____ **ACTIVITY # 74:** Associating Words
MATERIALS: a watch with a second hand, pencil, and paper
WHAT TO DO: Think of a category and tell the patient that he has one minute to name as many things as he can in that category. Keep track of the number of things he names.

EXAMPLE:
     If you say "things you could buy in a bakery"
then he names as many as he can in one minute.
     Continue with other categories.
VARIATION: You can keep track of the categories and how many he says in one minute. He can try to improve his score at another time.
SIMPLIFYING THE ACTIVITY: You can use broad categories that' provide a lot of possibilities from which to choose. Give a time limit from two to five minutes to name things.

_____ **ACTIVITY # 75:** Associating Words
MATERIALS: paper and pencil
WHAT TO DO: Think of a category and tell the patient what it is.
Name a letter and write it down. Ask him to name something in the
category that begins with that letter.

EXAMPLE:
    If you say "sports" and write the letter "s"
*then he can say "soccer," "skiing," "swimming," or another sport beginning
with "s."*
    If you say "states" and write the letter "C"
*then he can say "California," "Colorado," or another state beginning with
"C."*
    Continue with other categories.
VARIATION: Instead of changing categories, change the letters that
you use.
EXPANDING THE ACTIVITY: Ask the patient to name as many
things as he can think of in the category.

_____ **ACTIVITY # 76:** Associating a Letter
MATERIALS: paper and pencil
WHAT TO DO: Write the alphabet in capital letters. Choose a gen-
eral category and tell the patient what it is. Ask him to name some-
thing in that category that begins with each letter of the alphabet.
(You can skip Q, X, Y, and Z.)

EXAMPLE:
    Some categories include: foods, names, countries, occupations,
animals, cities, famous people, colors, vegetables.

_____ **ACTIVITY # 77:** Associating Familiar Words
MATERIALS: none
WHAT TO DO: Think of something familiar and tell the patient the
general category it is in. Ask him to guess what you are thinking of.

EXAMPLE:
    If you are thinking of *Time* magazine, then you can say the cate-
gory is "something you read" or "a magazine."
He guesses until he gets the correct answer.
    Continue by thinking of another item.
REMINDER: If the patient is having difficulty thinking of things, give
him a clue.

SIMPLIFYING THE ACTIVITY: Give the patient some clues before he starts guessing.

EXPANDING THE ACTIVITY: Name a very general category and don't offer any clues unless needed.

_____ **ACTIVITY # 78:** Identifying an Object
MATERIALS: none
WHAT TO DO: Ask questions about familiar things that the patient can answer in one word.

EXAMPLE:
   If you ask "what do you use to clean laundry?"
then he can say "soap," "washing machine," "detergent," or another correct answer.
   If you ask "what did you have for dessert today?"
then he says the correct answer.
   If you ask "what do you cook an egg in?"
then he says "pan" or another correct answer.
   Continue by asking other questions.

_____ **ACTIVITY # 79:** Identifying Facts
MATERIALS: none
WHAT TO DO: Ask factual questions about anything that the patient can answer in one word.

EXAMPLE:
   If you ask "in what month is Halloween?"
then he says "October."
   If you ask "where is London?"
then he says "England."
   Continue with other factual questions.

_____ **ACTIVITY # 80:** Identifying an Item
MATERIALS: a merchandise catalog (such as Sears), an advertising circular, a gift catalog or a brochure. It must have descriptions of the items for sale.
WHAT TO DO: Choose an item that can be purchased. Read a description of that item, but don't tell the patient what you are reading. Ask him to tell you what you have described.

EXAMPLE:

If you say "antique brass model. Thirteen inches high, shade has pleated fabric over it. Hi–lo dimmer switch. Takes 100-watt bulb" *then he says "lamp."*

Continue by describing other items.

REMINDER: Be careful not to mention the item in your description.

SIMPLIFYING THE ACTIVITY: If he cannot read, show him the page with the items. Ask him to point to the one he thinks you are describing.

EXPANDING THE ACTIVITY: Read one sentence at a time. Let the patient guess an item before you read further.

_____ **Activity # 81:** Naming

MATERIALS: none

WHAT TO DO: Your clinician has checked some examples to practice. Describe one of the items. Give enough clues so that it is not too hard to figure out what you are thinking.

EXAMPLE:

_____ Anything in the room

_____ Anything that could be in the house

_____ A place (city, country, state, monument, body of water, tourist attraction, etc.)

_____ A famous person (entertainer, actor, actress, politician, author, explorer, inventor, etc.)

_____ Any food

_____ Relatives or friends

_____ Any word you can describe (use a dictionary if needed)

_____ Hum a tune

_____ **ACTIVITY # 82:** Naming

MATERIALS: a dictionary or easy crossword puzzle

WHAT TO DO: Read a definition from either a dictionary or a crossword puzzle. Ask the patient to name the word you are describing.

EXAMPLE:

If you say "a piece of jewelry you wear on your finger" *then he says "ring."*

If you say "a five-sided figure" *then he says "pentagon."*

Continue with other definitions.

REMINDER: If the patient answers with a word which is reasonable, but is not the word you chose, it is still an acceptable answer.

SIMPLIFYING THE ACTIVITY: You can choose easier words. If he can read, you can put dashes on a sheet of paper to show how many letters are in the word, or you can write the first letter of the word.
EXPANDING THE ACTIVITY: Use more difficult examples.

——— **ACTIVITY # 83:** Naming Familiar Things
MATERIALS: a watch with a second hand
WHAT TO DO: Ask the patient to look around. Tell him he has two minutes to name as many different things as he can. Keep track of how many things he names.
VARIATION: Keep track of how many things he names, and compare this score to his score the next time.
SIMPLIFYING THE ACTIVITY: Time him for more than two minutes.
EXPANDING THE ACTIVITY: Time him for one minute only.

Other Activities

Talking

This section helps the patient use his speech skills. Since the patient may have difficulty saying more than one word or explaining a thought, these activities will provide practice in talking.

It is sometimes easier for the aphasic person to communicate in single words than in phrases or sentences. This is especially true if those around him anticipate his desires or fail to encourage him to speak whenever possible. It is important to create speaking situations for him. You might also ask him to repeat things if he is not able to speak on his own. Ask more questions than you would ordinarily. Try not to talk when he is trying to think, and even if he is having trouble, try not to fill in words for him or interrupt him.

The following kinds of activities are done in this section on Talking:

Answering Questions	Activities 84–85
Rewording	Activity 86
Completing Sentences	Activities 87–88
Constructing Sentences	Activities 89–91
Answering in Complete Sentences	Activities 92–93
Explaining Ideas	Activity 94
Asking Questions	Activities 95–98
Describing Things	Activities 99–103
Explaining Complex Ideas	Activities 104–9

Your speech-language pathologist will fill out this part.

Do _____ session(s) each day with the patient.

Do not spend any more than _____ minutes each session working.

_____ Correct any mistakes he makes.

_____ Do not correct his mistakes, but continue to the next question.

_____ Repeat the question if he makes a mistake.

_____ Keep track of any errors he makes.

_____ Do not keep track of his errors.

_____ Work on several activities at each working session.

_____ Work on only one activity during each working session.

Notes

_____ **ACTIVITY # 84:** Answering Questions
MATERIALS: none
WHAT TO DO: Make a short statement about something, then ask the patient a question about the statement.

EXAMPLE:
    If you say "I have a dog," pause, and ask "what do I have?"
then he says "a dog."
    If you say "the cheese is moldy," pause, and ask "what's the matter with the cheese?"
then he says "it's moldy."
    Continue by making other statements.

_____ **ACTIVITY # 85:** Answering Questions
MATERIALS: none
WHAT TO DO: Ask a simple yes-or-no question, which the patient should answer in a sentence.

EXAMPLE:
    If you ask "are you sitting down?"
then he says "yes, I am sitting down."

If you ask "is Paris in England?"
then he says "no, Paris is not in England."
If you ask "do you sleep in a bathtub?"
then he says "no, I don't sleep in a bathtub."
Continue with other questions.

REMINDER: If the answer to your question is no, he is to repeat the question in negative form, as the examples show. You can ask questions which have very obvious answers. The goal is for the patient to repeat your question using yes or no as part of his answer.

SIMPLIFYING THE ACTIVITY: If the patient cannot answer in a complete sentence, encourage him to repeat part of the sentence. You can say the answer for him and ask him to repeat it.

_____ **ACTIVITY # 86:** Rewording Sentences

MATERIALS: none

WHAT TO DO: Say a sentence which is not logical, with an incorrect word or idea. Ask the patient to change your sentence so that it makes sense.

EXAMPLE:
If you say "I keep ice cream in the stove"
then he says "I keep ice cream in the freezer."
If you say "you cut meat with a spoon"
then he says "you cut meat with a knife."
If you say "Babe Ruth was a famous musician"
then he says "Babe Ruth was a famous athlete" or "Beethoven was a famous musician."
Continue with other incorrect sentences.

REMINDER: All sentences should have a part that does not make sense. If you can't think of any, use sentences from a book or magazine and change a word or two.

SIMPLIFYING THE ACTIVITY: Use sentences which are about things the patient can see. For instance, your sentence can be "I am wearing a blue sweater," which he changes to "You are wearing a red sweater."

EXPANDING THE ACTIVITY: Use sentences which almost sound correct but are not. For instance, your sentence can be "I talked the dog around the block," which he changes to "I walked the dog around the block."

_____ **ACTIVITY # 87:** Completing Sentences

MATERIALS: none

WHAT TO DO: Say the first part of a sentence, then let the patient complete it in any way.

EXAMPLE:

If you say "I wish that . . ."
then he can say "it would stop raining," or "I had a million dollars," or any other ending that makes sense.

If you say "the guests were . . ."
then he can say "late for the party" or "talking on the patio," or any other ending that makes sense.

Continue with other first parts of sentences.

REMINDER: Encourage the patient to add as many words as he can.

SIMPLIFYING THE ACTIVITY: Use sentences in which only a word or two needs to be added to complete a thought.

_____ **ACTIVITY # 88:** Completing Sentences

MATERIALS: none

WHAT TO DO: Talk about an idea or short story, stop during the middle, and ask the patient to continue the idea. Encourage him to add as much as he would like to the story.

EXAMPLE:

If you say "It started out as a bad day. I couldn't find my slippers, I cut myself shaving, and that was just the beginning. I went into the kitchen and . . ."
then he continues the story in any way that makes sense.

If you say "There are several things to think about when you change a lightbulb. The first thing to do is . . ."
then he continues the idea in any way that makes sense.

Continue with other ideas for him to complete.

SIMPLIFYING THE ACTIVITY: End your sentence so that only a few words are added to make a complete thought. For instance, in the first example you can say "I walked into the kitchen and slipped on. . . ." Then he will only need to add a word or two, such as "some water," "a banana peel," "a piece of paper," etc.

_____ **ACTIVITY # 89:** Constructing Sentences

MATERIALS: none

WHAT TO DO: Say a word, then ask the patient to think of a sentence with that word in it. Ask him to say it out loud.

EXAMPLE:

If you say "apple"
then he can say "I ate an apple," "apples grow on trees," "I like apple cider," or another sentence that uses the word apple correctly.

If you say "open"

then he can say "please open the door," "the store will open at 9:00 A.M.," or another sentence using the word correctly.

Continue with other words for him to put in sentences.

SIMPLIFYING THE ACTIVITY: Choose words that name things (window, bread) or words that can begin a sentence (I, the, you).

EXPANDING THE ACTIVITY: Choose an idea which is more difficult to put into words, such as boredom, jealousy, or shyness.

_____ ACTIVITY # 90: Constructing Sentences

MATERIALS: none

WHAT TO DO: Say a phrase, then ask the patient to think of a sentence with that phrase in it. Ask him to say it out loud.

EXAMPLE:

If you say "not ready"

then he can say "the letter is not ready to be typed," or "I'm not ready to go out," or another sentence using the phrase correctly.

If you say "in the barn"

then he can say "the horses are in the barn," or "she went in the barn to find a rake," or another sentence using the phrase correctly.

Continue with other phrases for him to put in sentences.

REMINDER: You can use any phrase that you can think of or find in a newspaper or magazine.

_____ ACTIVITY # 91: Constructing Sentences

MATERIALS: none

WHAT TO DO: Tell the patient to watch you. Pretend you are doing some kind of movement or action by using your body and any props. Do not speak. Ask him to explain what you are doing.

EXAMPLE:

If you put your hands on your head

then he says "you put your hands on your head."

If you stand up and make motions like you are vacuuming a rug

then he says "you are using the vacuum."

If you pretend you are asleep

then he says "you are sleeping."

Continue with other actions.

REMINDER: Encourage him to answer in complete sentences.

VARIATION: This activity can be done throughout the day as you do different tasks. For instance, if you are making coffee, you can ask him to describe what you are doing as you go along.

SIMPLIFYING THE ACTIVITY: Let him tell you in a few words what you are doing. He does not have to answer in a complete sentence.
EXPANDING THE ACTIVITY: Pretend you are going through a series of actions but ask him to talk about what you are doing during each step. For instance, if you choose making a phone call, then the steps might be as follows: picking up the phone, dialing a number, talking, and hanging up the phone.

_____ **ACTIVITY # 92:** Answering in Complete Sentences
MATERIALS: none
WHAT TO DO: Ask the patient a question about something that happened or is going to happen during the day.

EXAMPLE:
   If you ask "did you get any mail?
then he answers.
   If you ask "what happened an hour ago?"
then he answers.
   Continue with other questions about his day.
REMINDER: Encourage him to answer in complete sentences. You can ask about something out of the ordinary (such as seeing a movie), something that happens every day (such as brushing teeth), or something more specific (such as naming what he ate).

_____ **ACTIVITY # 93:** Answering in Sentences
MATERIALS: none
WHAT TO DO: Ask the patient a question that requires a fairly short but complete answer.

EXAMPLE:
   If you ask "why do you brush your teeth?"
then he can say "I brush my teeth to clean my mouth," "I brush my teeth to prevent tooth decay," or another answer.
   If you say "who is Walter Cronkite?"
then he can say "reporter at six o'clock," "he was a news commentator for CBS," or another answer.
   Continue with other questions.
REMINDER: Encourage him to answer in complete sentences. You can ask any questions just so a long answer is not required.
SIMPLIFYING THE ACTIVITY: Let him answer in a few words rather than a complete sentence.
EXPANDING THE ACTIVITY: Ask him to answer in complete sentences with as much information as possible.

_____ **ACTIVITY # 94:** Explaining Ideas
MATERIALS: none
WHAT TO DO: Say a word, then ask the patient to explain what the word means. Choose a word that is not too hard to define.

EXAMPLE:
    If you ask "what is an eraser?"
then he can say "it's for getting rid of mistakes," or "you use it when you goof," or "it fixes things when you write," or another correct answer.
    If you ask "what does the word continue mean?"
then he can say "on and on," "keep going," or another correct answer.
    Continue with other words to explain.
REMINDER: If he puts the word in a sentence but does not tell what it means, ask him again. Emphasize that you want him to explain the meaning.
SIMPLIFYING THE ACTIVITY: Let him answer in a few words rather than a complete sentence.
EXPANDING THE ACTIVITY: Use words that might be a little harder to define. You can use a dictionary to help find them.

_____ **ACTIVITY # 95:** Asking Questions
MATERIALS: none
WHAT TO DO: Make a short statement, then tell the patient to ask you a question about your statement.

EXAMPLE:
    If you say "I am wearing brown shoes"
then he can ask "what color shoes are you wearing?"; "are you wearing green shoes?" or "are you wearing boots?"
    If you say "the letter is on the table"
then he can ask "is the letter on the floor?"; "where is the letter?"; or "what is on the table?"
    Continue with other statements.

_____ **ACTIVITY # 96:** Asking Questions
MATERIALS: action pictures (see Appendix C)
WHAT TO DO: Place a picture on the table, and tell the patient to ask you a question about the picture.

EXAMPLE:
    If the picture shows a man holding a large fish
then he can ask questions like "what is the man holding?"; "what color is the man's shirt?"; or "how does the man feel?"

Replace the picture with another one and continue.

VARIATION: He can ask you several questions about each picture.

SIMPLIFYING THE ACTIVITY: You can suggest that he start his question by using one of the following words: who, what, when, where, or how. If he has difficulty choosing one of these, then help him by giving him a word or two to begin his sentence.

_____ **ACTIVITY # 97:** Asking Questions

MATERIALS: none

WHAT TO DO: Make any statement and tell the patient to ask you a question about your statement.

EXAMPLE:

If you say "I am tired today"

then he can ask "why are you tired?"; "were you tired yesterday?"; or "do you feel tired?"

If you say "porcupines have long quills"

then he can ask "what has long quills?"; "do porcupines have short quills?"; or "what are quills?"

Continue with other statements.

VARIATION: You can use action pictures (see Appendix C). Choose a picture and tell the patient to ask you a question about the picture.

_____ **ACTIVITY # 98:** Asking Questions

MATERIALS: none

WHAT TO DO: You are going to think of something, and the patient is going to guess what you are thinking. Give him a clue about what you picked, such as a person, place, thing, animal, vegetable, mineral, etc. Tell him to ask you questions to help him figure out what you have chosen.

EXAMPLE:

If you choose a clock, your clue can be that it is found in any room of the house.

Then he can ask questions such as "is it bigger than a breadbox?" or "is there one in this room?"

He guesses until he thinks of a clock.

Continue with something else for him to guess.

REMINDER: Encourage the patient to ask questions which will provide information to help him, rather than just guessing at random.

SIMPLIFYING THE ACTIVITY: Give him some more information before he starts asking you questions. Let him guess some specific things in addition to asking questions.

EXPANDING THE ACTIVITY: Limit the number of questions he can ask you.

_____ **ACTIVITY # 99:** Describing Things
MATERIALS: pictures of objects (see Appendix B)
WHAT TO DO: Place a picture on the table, and ask the patient to explain what you can do with that item.

EXAMPLE:
Suppose a picture of a suitcase is on the table.
If you ask "what is a suitcase used for?"
then he can say "you can use it to carry clothes" or another correct sentence.
Suppose a picture of a watch is on the table.
If you ask "what do you do with a watch?"
then he can say "it tells time," "a watch gives you the time of day," or another correct sentence.
Change pictures and continue with more questions.
REMINDER: Encourage him to speak in complete sentences.
VARIATION: Use small objects (see Appendix A) instead of pictures.
SIMPLIFYING THE ACTIVITY: Let him answer in a few words rather than in complete sentences.

_____ **ACTIVITY # 100:** Describing Things
MATERIALS: small objects (see Appendix A)
WHAT TO DO: Place an object on the table, and ask the patient to describe it. Encourage him to make the description as complete as possible.

EXAMPLE:
If a lemon is on the table
then he can say "it's a fruit," "it's yellow," "it's sour," "you eat it," "it's smaller than an orange," "it's citrus," etc.
Replace the object with a different one and continue.
REMINDER: You might have to ask questions about the item to get him started. You can ask him to talk about the following: size, shape, color, where it comes from, what it is made of, how it is used, etc. Encourage him to use complete sentences.
VARIATION: You can use pictures of objects (see Appendix B) instead of the objects themselves. You can tell him not to show you the object—you can guess what it is.
SIMPLIFYING THE ACTIVITY: He can describe it in a few words rather than complete sentences. You can ask him questions about the item's size, shape, color, etc.

_____ ACTIVITY # 101: Describing Things
MATERIALS: action pictures (see Appendix C)
WHAT TO DO: Place a picture on the table, and ask the patient to describe what is happening in it.

EXAMPLE:
Suppose the picture shows a man walking out of a grocery store holding a bag.
He can say such things as "the man is leaving the store," "he just got some groceries," "it looks like the bag is heavy and the man is going to fall if he doesn't look out," or other correct sentences.
Replace the picture with a different one and continue.
SIMPLIFYING THE ACTIVITY: Let him answer in a few words rather than a complete sentence.
EXPANDING THE ACTIVITY: Encourage him to talk about the picture in detail or to make up a story about the picture.

_____ ACTIVITY # 102: Describing Things
MATERIALS: family photographs
WHAT TO DO: Place a photo on the table, and ask the patient to tell you what he knows about the photo, such as where it was taken, when it was taken, who is in the picture, why it was taken, etc.

EXAMPLE:
Suppose the picture shows a small child in front of a big cake.
He can say "she's my granddaughter," "Judy was three years old," "we had a birthday party for Judy," "this was taken two years ago at Bob and Carol's," or other correct sentences.
Replace the picture with a different one and continue.
REMINDER: Encourage him to give you as much information as possible.
SIMPLIFYING THE ACTIVITY: Let him explain in a few words rather than complete sentences.

_____ ACTIVITY # 103: Describing Things
MATERIALS: none
WHAT TO DO: Ask the patient to think of a person, a place, an animal, a food, a TV show, or a movie and to describe it in complete sentences using as much detail as possible. When he finishes, you are to guess what he is talking about. If you think he can add more to his description, ask him questions to give you more information.

EXAMPLE:

If the patient says "I'm thinking of a man. He was president during the Civil War. He was tall. He had a beard. He was shot, and he wrote the Gettysburg Address"
then you guess "Abraham Lincoln."

If he says "it's a place in the U.S. People go there for honeymoons. It's between New York and Canada. It has lots of water and rocks. It has lots of tourists"
then you guess "Niagara Falls."

Continue by having him describe other things.

REMINDER: Encourage him to use a lot of description.

SIMPLIFYING THE ACTIVITY: Let him describe what he is thinking of in a few words rather than in complete sentences.

_____ **ACTIVITY # 104:** Explaining Ideas

MATERIALS: none

WHAT TO DO: Think of something that takes several steps to complete, and ask the patient to explain step by step how it would be done.

EXAMPLE:

If you ask "how do you brush your teeth?"
then he can say "you get out a toothbrush. Put toothpaste on it. Put it in your mouth and brush. Rinse your mouth. Put it away."
If you ask "how do you use a charge card?"
then he can say "take the things you want to the cash register. Get out the card. Say 'charge it.' The clerk puts the card in a machine and gives you a paper. Sign your name and don't forget the card."

Continue by asking him to explain other things.

REMINDER: Encourage him to use complete sentences.

SIMPLIFYING THE ACTIVITY: Ask him to tell you the first thing to do (he tells you), then the next thing (he tells you), then the next, etc. Take one step at a time.

_____ **ACTIVITY # 105:** Explaining Ideas

MATERIALS: a map

WHAT TO DO: Take a map of an area and open it on the table. Point to two places on the map, and ask the patient to explain how to get from one place to the other.

EXAMPLE:

Suppose a map of New York is on the table. If you point to Buffalo and Albany
then he tells you what roads or routes to take to get from one city to the other.

REMINDER: Encourage him to give directions in complete sentences.
VARIATION: You can write down the directions as he gives them, then read them aloud as he uses his finger to check his route.
SIMPLIFYING THE ACTIVITY: You can use a map of a familiar area. You can use a map with just a few lines, such as one in a newspaper or in a brochure showing the location of a store. You can put a mark somewhere on that map and ask him to direct you from there to the store.

—— **ACTIVITY # 106:** Explaining Ideas
MATERIALS: none
WHAT TO DO: Using the three basic parts of a conversation, practice talking, listening, and asking questions. Begin a conversation with the patient by asking him questions to encourage him to talk. When he is finished, let him question you. Encourage him to ask several questions.

EXAMPLE:
   Some conversation starters include people in the news, the plot of a TV show, politics, work, friends, current events, nutrition, health, crafts, hobbies, cars, sports.
REMINDER: Some people are not "talkers" and may have trouble getting started. Choose a subject that might be of particular interest to that person.

—— **ACTIVITY # 107:** Explaining Ideas
MATERIALS: none
WHAT TO DO: Pick a topic about which there can be opposite points of view. State one view and ask the patient to talk about a different viewpoint.

EXAMPLE:
   If you say "I think murder and violence on TV are good things" *then he takes an opposite point of view. He can say "I think it's bad because kids can watch the shows and that's not good for them. They could get bad ideas."*
   Continue with other topics.
REMINDER: Encourage the patient to talk in complete sentences. Remember that neither of you has to talk about your own feelings, but that he is to take an opposite view from what you have stated.
SIMPLIFYING THE ACTIVITY: Let him answer in a few words rather than complete sentences. If you know his point of view, take the opposite one, so that he will be expressing his own opinion.

EXPANDING THE ACTIVITY: Choose a subject. Ask him to talk about one point of view. When he finishes, ask him to talk about the opposite point of view. For instance, if you ask him to talk about cigarette smoking, he can tell you its pros and cons.

_____ **ACTIVITY # 108:** Explaining Ideas
MATERIALS: a television set
WHAT TO DO: Watch a TV show with the patient. After it is over, ask him to explain what happened. Encourage him to give as much detail as he can.

EXAMPLE:
        If you watch a movie, drama, situation comedy, or soap opera
then he can talk about the plot and explain the story as it happened.
        If you watch an entertainment or talk show
then he can talk about who the guests were, what they did, and the different things that happened on the show.
        If you watch an educational or news show
then he can talk about what he learned or what he heard.
REMINDER: Encourage him to talk in complete sentences.
SIMPLIFYING THE ACTIVITY: Let him explain in a few words rather than complete sentences. You can ask questions about some things you saw or about different things that happened on the show. You can ask him to talk about one part of the program. You can ask him yes-or-no questions that he can answer by nodding or shaking his head.

_____ **ACTIVITY # 109:** Explaining Ideas
MATERIALS: none
WHAT TO DO: Your clinician has checked some examples to practice. Ask the patient to explain them to you. If he has difficulty thinking of a specific idea, suggest one. If he has difficulty staying on a topic or putting his thoughts together in the right order, ask questions to help him.

EXAMPLE:
_____ Jokes
_____ Stories
_____ Recalling things that happened when he was younger
_____ Vacation or travel stories
_____ Recalling special events in his life
_____ Explaining how to play a game
REMINDER: Encourage him to talk in complete sentences. He

doesn't need to mention every detail, but you ought to be able to understand what he is talking about.

SIMPLIFYING THE ACTIVITY: Choose one of the topics, remind him of a specific idea, and ask him to tell you about it. Ask questions to help him with his story if he needs it.

Other Activities

Memory

This section concerns itself with activities for memory. In general there are two kinds of memory: the ability to recall events or facts from the past (yesterday, last week, or ten years ago), and the ability to remember things we have just heard and need understand only long enough to react to them.

Most of this section has activities for reacting to things just heard. There are also some activities to test the ability to recall older events or facts. Most activities do not require any speaking ability on the part of the patient.

The following kinds of activities are done in this section on Memory:

Following Directions	Activities 110, 119, 121, 129
Remembering Words	Activities 111–12, 125–26, 130
Recalling Information	Activities 113–17, 127–28, 131–35
Remembering Objects	Activities 114–16, 118, 120, 122–24

Your speech-language pathologist will fill out this part.

Do _____ session(s) each day with the patient.

Do not spend any more than _____ minutes each session working.

_____ Correct any mistakes he makes.

_____ Do not correct his mistakes, but continue to the next question.

_____ Repeat the question if he makes a mistake.

_____ Keep track of any errors he makes.

_____ Do not keep track of his errors.

_____Workon several activities at each working session.

_____. Work on only one activity during each working session.

Notes

_____ **ACTIVITY # 110:** Following Directions
MATERIALS: none
WHAT TO DO: Name two parts of the body, and ask the patient to
point to them in the order in which you named them.

EXAMPLE:
If you say "point to your elbow and your waist"
then he points first to his elbow and then to his waist.
If you say "point to your knee and your hair"
then he points to them in order.
Continue by asking him to point to other parts of his body.
REMINDER: Have the patient wait until you name both body parts
before he starts to point. Have him point to them in the proper
order.
EXPANDING THE ACTIVITY: Ask him to point to three body
parts instead of two, and continue as before. If his answers remain
correct, add a fourth body part. Add more body parts until he has
difficulty.

_____ **ACTIVITY # 111:** Remembering Words in Order
MATERIALS: none
WHAT TO DO: Name two things in the room for the patient to
locate, and ask him to point to these things in the order in which you
said them.

EXAMPLE:
If you ask "where are the telephone and the doorknob?"
then he points to them in that order.
If you say "where is the light and the newspaper?"
then he points to them in that order.
Continue by naming two other things in the room.
REMINDER: Look at the patient and not at the objects when you
talk. Have him wait until you name both things before he starts to
point.
VARIATION: He can go over and touch the things you mention instead of pointing to them.
EXPANDING THE ACTIVITY: Ask him to point to three things
instead of two, and continue as before. If his answers remain correct,
add a fourth thing. Add more things until he has difficulty.

_____ **ACTIVITY # 112:** Remembering Words in Order
MATERIALS: small objects (see Appendix A)
WHAT TO DO: Place five objects on the table, and name any three.

Ask the patient to point to the ones that you named in the order in which you named them.

EXAMPLE:

Suppose these objects are on the table: a spool of thread, a spoon, a penny, a watch, and a toothbrush.

If you say "thread, spoon, and watch"
then he points to them in that order.

If you say "penny, thread, toothbrush"
then he points to them in that order.

Replace two of the objects with different ones and continue.

REMINDER: The patient is to wait until you name all three objects before he starts to point.

VARIATION: You can use any of the following: pictures of objects (see Appendix B), a deck of playing cards (name the cards for him), or coupons (name the product).

SIMPLIFYING THE ACTIVITY: Place four objects on the table instead of five. Ask him to point to two of them.

EXPANDING THE ACTIVITY: Place six objects on the table instead of five, and continue as before. If his answers remain correct, add a seventh object and have him point to four in order. If his answers are still correct, add an eighth object and have him point to five in order. Add more objects until he has difficulty.

—— **ACTIVITY # 113:** Remembering Ideas

MATERIALS: small objects (see Appendix A)

WHAT TO DO: Place five objects on the table. Describe the use of two of the objects, and ask the patient to point to those objects in the order in which you described them.

EXAMPLE:

Suppose these objects are on the table: a salt shaker, a pencil, a can opener, a deck of playing cards, and a scissors.

If you say "point to the one you use to write and the one you use to cut"
then he points to the pencil and scissors in that order.

If you say "point to the one you use on food and the one you need for gin rummy"
then he points to the salt shaker and the cards in that order.

Replace two of the objects with different ones and continue.

REMINDER: Have him wait until you describe all the objects before he starts to point.

VARIATION: Use pictures of objects (see Appendix B) or photographs instead of real objects.

SIMPLIFYING THE ACTIVITY: Place three or four objects on the table instead of five.

EXPANDING THE ACTIVITY: Place six objects on the table instead of five, and continue as before. If his answers remain correct, add a seventh object and describe four things for him to point to in order. Add more objects until he has difficulty.

———— **ACTIVITY # 114:** Remembering What You See

MATERIALS: pictures of objects (see Appendix B)

WHAT TO DO: Place three pictures on the table and tell the patient to look at them and think about what they are. When he is ready, tell him to close his eyes. Remove one of the pictures, then ask him to open his eyes and tell you which one is missing.

EXAMPLE:

Suppose pictures of a car, some meat, and a bear are on the table. When he closes his eyes, remove a picture.

If you remove the picture of the meat

then he opens his eyes and tells you that the meat picture is missing.

If you remove the picture of the car

then he opens his eyes and tells you that the car picture is missing.

Replace two of the pictures with different ones and continue.

REMINDER: If he cannot keep his eyes closed, put a piece of cardboard or a box lid in front of the pictures when you remove them.

VARIATION: You can use any of the following: small objects (see Appendix A), photographs, a deck of playing cards, or coupons.

EXPANDING THE ACTIVITY: Place four pictures on the table instead of three, and continue as before. If his answers remain correct, then add a fifth picture. Add more pictures until he has difficulty. If his answers still remain correct, remove two pictures instead of one.

———— **ACTIVITY # 115:** Remembering What You See

MATERIALS: pictures of objects (see Appendix B)

WHAT TO DO: Place three pictures on the table and tell the patient to look at them and think about their order. When he is ready, tell him to close his eyes. Rearrange the pictures, then ask him to open his eyes and put them back in their original order.

EXAMPLE:

Suppose these pictures are on the table: a glass on the left, a nail file in the middle, and a ring on the right. After he closes his eyes, rearrange them.

If you put the file on the left, the glass in the middle, and the ring on the right
then he puts them back in their original order.
Replace one of the pictures with a different one and continue.
REMINDER: If he cannot keep his eyes closed, put a piece of cardboard or a box lid in front of the pictures while you rearrange them.
VARIATION: You can use any of the following: photographs, a deck of playing cards, coupons, or credit cards.
EXPANDING THE ACTIVITY: Place four pictures on the table instead of three, and continue as before. If his answers remain correct, then add a fifth picture. Add more pictures until he has difficulty.

_____ **ACTIVITY # 116:** Remembering What You See
MATERIALS: pictures of objects (see Appendix B) and a box lid or a piece of cardboard
WHAT TO DO: Place three pictures on the table and ask the patient to look at them and think about what they are. When he is ready, cover the pictures with the cardboard or the box lid, then ask him what the pictures are.

EXAMPLE:
Suppose these pictures are on the table: a towel, a vase, and a TV. When he is ready, put the lid or cardboard in front of them. Then ask him to name the pictures you have covered.
He says, "towel, vase, and TV."
Replace the pictures with different ones and continue.
VARIATION: Use small objects (see Appendix A).
SIMPLIFYING THE ACTIVITY: Place two pictures on the table instead of three.
EXPANDING THE ACTIVITY: Place four pictures on the table instead of three, and continue as before. If his answers remain correct, then add a fifth picture. Add more pictures until he has difficulty.

_____ **ACTIVITY # 117:** Remembering Ideas
MATERIALS: pictures of objects (see Appendix B)
WHAT TO DO: Give the patient three pictures. Have him put them on the table in a certain order, but ask him to wait until you finish talking before he puts any pictures down.

EXAMPLE:
Suppose he has these pictures: a pair of shoes, a bed, and a stove.
If you say "put the stove, bed, and shoes on the table in that order"

then he does it.

Continue by giving him three more pictures.

REMINDER: Have him wait until you name all three pictures before he starts.

VARIATION: Use a deck of playing cards.

EXPANDING THE ACTIVITY: Give him four pictures to put on the table instead of three, and continue as before. If his answers remain correct, then add a fifth picture. Add more pictures until he has difficulty.

_____ **ACTIVITY # 118:** Remembering What You See
MATERIALS: none
WHAT TO DO: Make two different movements, then ask the patient to imitate what you did in the same order.

EXAMPLE:

If you point to your knee and then your throat
then he points to his knee and throat in that order.

Continue with other movements.

REMINDER: Have him wait until you make both movements before he starts.

EXPANDING THE ACTIVITY: Make three movements instead of two.

_____ **ACTIVITY # 119:** Following Directions
MATERIALS: none
WHAT TO DO: Give the patient two directions to follow.

EXAMPLE:

If you ask him to make a fist, then cross his arms
he does it in that order.

If you ask him to put his left hand on his right shoulder, then count backwards from five
he does it in that order.

Continue by giving him other directions.

REMINDER: Have him wait until you give both directions before he starts.

EXPANDING THE ACTIVITY: Give him three directions instead of two.

_____ **ACTIVITY # 120:** Remembering What You See
MATERIALS: small objects (see Appendix A)
WHAT TO DO: Place five objects on the table in a particular ar-

rangement. Tell the patient to look at the arrangement and remember it. Then give him the objects and ask him to arrange them exactly as you had them.

EXAMPLE:
Suppose these objects are on the table: a roll of scotch tape on its side, a necklace in a small box, and a key wrapped in a napkin. When he is ready, pick up the objects and put them in front of him in a pile. Ask him to put the objects back on the table the way they were. *Then he does it.*

Replace one of the objects with another one, make a different arrangement, and continue.
SIMPLIFYING THE ACTIVITY: Use three objects instead of five, and continue as before. If his answers remain correct, use four objects.
EXPANDING THE ACTIVITY: Use six objects instead of five, and continue as before. If his answers remain correct, use seven objects instead of six.

_____ ACTIVITY # 121: Remembering Directions
MATERIALS: small objects (see Appendix A)
WHAT TO DO: Place four objects in a line on the table, and give the patient two directions to follow.

EXAMPLE:
Suppose these objects are on the table: a comb, a ruler, a light bulb, and a stick of gum.
If you say "put the light bulb next to the comb and put the gum on the ruler"
then he does it.
If you say "turn over the stick of gum and hand me the comb"
then he does it.
Replace two of the objects with different ones and continue.
REMINDER: Have him wait until you give both directions before he starts.
SIMPLIFYING THE ACTIVITY: Use three objects instead of four.
EXPANDING THE ACTIVITY: Place five objects on the table instead of four, and continue as before. If his answers remain correct, then add a fifth object. Add more objects until he has difficulty.

_____ ACTIVITY # 122: Remembering What You See
MATERIALS: unlined paper, a felt-tip pen, a pencil
WHAT TO DO: Draw a simple design using shapes, lines, letters, numbers, etc. Tell the patient to look at the design and remember it.

When he is ready, cover it and ask him to draw the design from memory.

EXAMPLE:
Draw a square next to a circle and put a line under both of them, then let the patient look at it. When he is ready, cover it up *then he draws the same thing from memory.*
Draw the letter F and put a square around it and a star below the square, then let him look at it. When he is ready, cover it up *then he draws the same thing from memory.*
Continue by drawing different designs.
SIMPLIFYING THE ACTIVITY: Make your design more complicated by adding lines, shapes, etc.

_____ **ACTIVITY # 123:** Remembering What You See
MATERIALS: action pictures (see Appendix C)
WHAT TO DO: Place a picture on the table. Tell the patient to look at it and remember it. When he is ready, remove the picture and ask him to tell you everything he remembers about it.

EXAMPLE:
Suppose the picture is an advertisement and shows two people drinking wine in front of a fireplace. When he is ready, remove the picture and ask him to tell you what he remembers about it.
He can talk about what the people are wearing, what the fireplace looks like, what other things are in the picture, what the people look like, what they are doing, and any other details that he remembers.
Continue by showing him another picture.
SIMPLIFYING THE ACTIVITY: Ask him yes or no questions that he can answer by nodding or shaking his head.
EXPANDING THE ACTIVITY: Choose pictures that show a lot of activity.

_____ **ACTIVITY # 124:** Remembering What You See
MATERIALS: twenty pictures of objects (see Appendix B) and a piece of cardboard or a box lid
WHAT TO DO: Place the twenty pictures on the table in front of the patient. Tell him to look at them and think about what they are. Indicate that you are going to cover the pictures and then ask him to name as many as possible. When he is ready, place the cardboard box or lid over the pictures. As he names a picture, put it in front of him. When he names all that he can, remove the cover, and let him look at

the remaining pictures. When he is ready, again cover these pictures and ask him to name as many as he can, just as he did before.

Continue until he has named all of the pictures.

REMINDER: He is not expected to be able to remember all twenty pictures the first time.

VARIATION: Use small objects (see Appendix A) and cover them with a towel so that he will be able to see some of the shapes.

SIMPLIFYING THE ACTIVITY: Use ten pictures instead of twenty.

_____ **ACTIVITY # 125:** Remembering Words in Order

MATERIALS: none

WHAT TO DO: Say four words which are alike in some way. Do not use a sentence—just four separate words. Ask the patient to repeat the words in the order in which you said them.

EXAMPLE:

If you say "Eisenhower, Ford, Carter, Kennedy"
then he says them in the same order.

If you say "football, baseball, tennis ball, basketball"
then he says them in the same order.

Continue with other words.

VARIATION: Use four words from a list, such as an index, recipe ingredients, word search puzzle words, package ingredients, etc.

SIMPLIFYING THE ACTIVITY: Say three words instead of four.

EXPANDING THE ACTIVITY: Say five words instead of four, and continue as before. If his answers remain correct, then add a sixth word. Add more words until he has difficulty.

_____ **ACTIVITY # 126:** Remembering Words in Order

MATERIALS: none

WHAT TO DO: Say four words in a row. Do not use a sentence—just four separate words. Tell the patient to repeat the words in the order in which you said them.

EXAMPLE:

Suppose the words you say are "book, pen, apple, and snow."

If you ask "what was the last word I said?"
he says "snow."

If you ask "what was the second word?"
then he says "pen."

If you ask "what was the first word?"
then he says "book."

Continue with four more words.

REMINDER: Change the order in which you ask for answers so that he cannot memorize a pattern.

VARIATION: Use numbers instead of words.

SIMPLIFYING THE ACTIVITY: Use three words instead of four.

EXPANDING THE ACTIVITY: Use five words instead of four, and continue as before. If his answers remain correct, then add a sixth word. Add more words until he has difficulty.

_____ **ACTIVITY # 127:** Remembering Ideas

MATERIALS: none

WHAT TO DO: Tell the patient to listen while you say one or two sentences. Pause, then ask him questions about what you said.

EXAMPLE:

Suppose your sentences were: "Jane Jones went to the supermarket. She bought eggs, ginger ale, and oatmeal cookies."

If you ask "where did the lady go?"

then he says "the supermarket."

If you ask "what did she buy?"

then he says "eggs, ginger ale, and oatmeal cookies."

If you ask "what was her name?"

then he says "Jane Jones."

Continue with other sentences and questions.

REMINDER: You can use sentences from magazines or books. Any type of sentence that gives information may be used.

SIMPLIFYING THE ACTIVITY: Ask him yes-or-no questions that he can answer by nodding or shaking his head.

_____ **ACTIVITY # 128:** Remembering Sentences

MATERIALS: any reading material which gives information. If the material is longer than a paragraph, then choose one paragraph.

WHAT TO DO: Choose a paragraph and read it to the patient. Explain before you start that you will be asking him questions about the information that he is going to hear. When you finish reading, ask him questions about what you read.

REMINDER: Encourage him to answer in sentences. If he cannot, ask him questions which he can answer in a few words.

SIMPLIFYING THE ACTIVITY: Ask him yes-or-no questions that he can answer by nodding or shaking his head.

EXPANDING THE ACTIVITY: You can ask him to explain what he heard in his own words. If he leaves out some important facts, then ask him questions about them. You can also use longer paragraphs or use two or more paragraphs at one time.

_____ **ACTIVITY # 129:** Following Directions
MATERIALS: a map showing routes or streets and a toothpick
WHAT TO DO: Open the map so that a part of it is in front of the
patient. Trace a certain route aloud using the toothpick. After you
finish, ask him to retrace your route exactly as you did it. He can say
it out loud or trace it with the toothpick.

Continue by tracing other routes on the map.
REMINDER: If you do not have a detailed street map, you can use a
state map.
VARIATION: Look at the map and give your directions out loud but
do not trace the route. Ask him to repeat the directions.
SIMPLIFYING THE ACTIVITY: Make the directions simple and
choose a route between two places which are familiar to the patient.

_____ **ACTIVITY # 130:** Remembering Words in Order
MATERIALS: none
WHAT TO DO: Think of a category and tell the patient what it is. Say a
word in the category. He says your word, then adds a word of his own.
You say your first word, then his word, then add another word. Then he
says your first word, his word, and the third word (yours), and adds
another word of his own. Continue adding words and repeating them
until one of you cannot remember all of the words. Each word should
belong in the general category that you chose.

EXAMPLE:
Suppose you choose the category "furniture."
If you say "chair"
then he says "chair," and adds "table."
If you say "chair, table," and add "dresser"
then he says "chair, table, dresser," and adds another word.

Continue adding words until one of you cannot repeat them all.
Then begin a new category.
REMINDER: This activity can be done with several people. Each per-
son takes a turn and adds a word.
VARIATION: There are several variations to this activity. Your clini-
cian may have checked some of those below.

_____ Use words that begin with each letter of the alphabet. The
first word will begin with A, the second with B, etc.

_____ Start with any word. The next word will begin with the same
letter that the first word ends with. If the first word is "cat"
the next word has to start with "t."

_____ Use words that begin with one letter of the alphabet. If the
first word is "sun" then the rest of the words will begin with
the letter s.

_____ Each time begin with "I'm going on a trip and I'm going to take. . . ." You can name anything to take or you can name things in alphabetical order.

_____ Each time begin with "I'm going to the store and I'm going to buy. . . ." You can name anything to take or you can name things in alphabetical order.

_____ Each time begin with "I'm taking a trip and I'm going to visit. . . ." You can name any place or you can name places in alphabetical order.

_____ **ACTIVITY # 131:** Remembering Ideas

MATERIALS: see below

WHAT TO DO: Your clinician has checked some examples to practice. Read one of them, then ask the patient to tell you all that he remembers from what you read.

EXAMPLE:

_____ Descriptions in a catalog, flyer, magazine, etc.

_____ Descriptions of trips, publications, special offers, etc.

_____ Paragraphs in letters, newspapers, magazines, ads, books, etc.

_____ Labels or warranties on products

_____ Package directions, especially on foods

_____ Descriptions of courses in schools or colleges

_____ Lists of ingredients on products

_____ Directions from games

_____ Descriptions of houses for sale

_____ Individual want ads or classified ads

_____ Advertisements for products in newspapers, magazines, junk mail, etc.

_____ Descriptions of movies or TV shows

_____ Short articles in newspapers, magazines, etc.

SIMPLIFYING THE ACTIVITY: Ask yes-or-no questions that he can answer by nodding or shaking his head.

_____ **ACTIVITY # 132:** Remembering Ideas

MATERIALS: There are phone services which play a tape-recorded message. The list below provides examples of recorded messages for your area. Your clinician has either checked some messages available in your area or has added some. You will need a telephone and the telephone numbers to get the messages.

WHAT TO DO: Dial a message. Have the patient listen to the taped message and, when he is through, ask him questions about what he heard.

EXAMPLE:
_____ Time
_____ Weather
_____ Children's stories
_____ Lottery numbers
_____ Sports scores
_____ Movie theater information
_____ Medical information
_____ Consumer tips
_____ Entertainment information
_____ Horoscopes-by-Phone
_____ Thought for the day
_____ Dial-a-joke
_____ Soap Scoops

REMINDER: Some of the calls may be free, others not. The messages can usually be heard over and over, so if the patient doesn't understand the first time, he can keep listening.

SIMPLIFYING THE ACTIVITY: Ask him yes-or-no questions that he can answer by nodding or shaking his head.

EXPANDING THE ACTIVITY: Give him the phone number and have him dial it himself.

_____ **ACTIVITY # 133:** Recalling Past Information

MATERIALS: none

WHAT TO DO: Ask the patient questions using familiar information about himself and his environment.

EXAMPLE:
   If you ask "where are you?"
then he tells you.
   If you ask "what year is it?"
then he tells you.
   Continue with other questions.

_____ **ACTIVITY # 134:** Recalling Past Information

MATERIALS: none

WHAT TO DO: Ask the patient personal questions related to things that family members would know.

EXAMPLE:
   If you ask "at what bank do you have a checking account?"
then he answers correctly.

If you ask "what kind of car do you have?"
then he answers correctly.
Continue with other personal questions.
REMINDER: Questions can be about people, possessions, insurance, dates, places, etc.

_____ **ACTIVITY # 135:** Recalling Past Information
MATERIALS: none
WHAT TO DO: Ask the patient about things that have happened in his past (in the last half hour, the day before, the month before, etc.). Do not ask about specific dates, only general information.

EXAMPLE:
If you ask "what did you have for lunch?"
then he answers correctly.
If you ask "last week we celebrated a holiday and went some-where for dinner. Where did we go?"
then he tells you.
Continue with other questions.
SIMPLIFYING THE ACTIVITY: Explain a situation by setting the scene for him. Remind him of the details, then ask him a question about something you did not mention. For instance, if he can't remember what he had for lunch, you can remind him where he was eating, some of the things he was eating, and what else was on the table, or you can describe a certain food and ask him to tell you what it was.
EXPANDING THE ACTIVITY: Remind him of a situation and ask him to tell you as much about it as he can remember.

_____ **ACTIVITY # 136:** Recalling Past Information
MATERIALS: none
WHAT TO DO: Ask the patient general, factual questions which should be common knowledge.

EXAMPLE:
If you ask "how many things are in a dozen?"
then he says "twelve."
If you ask "who is the President of the United States?"
then he answers correctly.
If you ask "where is San Francisco?"
then he says "California."
Continue with other questions.

Other Activities

Spelling

One needs to be able to spell words before one can form a sentence. This section has activities which deal with recognizing and writing letters and spelling words.

The following kinds of activities are done in this section on Spelling:

Your speech-language pathologist will fill out this part.

Do _____ session(s) each day with the patient.

Do not spend any more than _____ minutes each session working.

_____ Correct any mistakes he makes.

_____ Do not correct his mistakes, but continue to the next question.

_____ Repeat the question if he makes a mistake.

_____ Keep track of any errors he makes.

_____ Do not keep track of his errors.

_____ Work on several activities at each working session.

_____ Work on only one activity during each working session.

Notes

_____ **ACTIVITY # 137:** Matching Letters
MATERIALS: word search puzzles, pen, and scrap paper
WHAT TO DO: Print a letter on a small sheet of paper. Ask the patient to look through a word search puzzle and mark that letter every time he sees it.

EXAMPLE:
　　If you print "e" on the paper
then he marks every "e" that he sees in the puzzle.
　　Continue by asking him to mark the letter by circling it, underlining it, or blackening it.
VARIATION: Print two letters on the paper and ask the patient to find both letters as he looks through the puzzle.
EXPANDING THE ACTIVITY: Have him look for several letters at one time.

_____ **ACTIVITY # 138:** Matching Letters
MATERIALS: paper and pencil and any printed material one can mark up (a newspaper, a magazine, a piece of junk mail, etc.)
WHAT TO DO: Choose some printed material and put it on the table. Print a letter on a small sheet of paper and ask the patient to mark that letter every time he sees it.

EXAMPLE:
　　If you choose a "Dear Abby" column and print the letter "t" on the paper
then he looks through the article and marks every "t" that he finds.
　　Continue with other letters and printed material.
REMINDER: The patient can mark the letter by circling it, crossing it out, underlining it, or blackening it.
VARIATION: Print two letters on the paper and ask him to find both letters.
SIMPLIFYING THE ACTIVITY: Use a short paragraph.
EXPANDING THE ACTIVITY: Use several paragraphs.

_____ **ACTIVITY # 139:** Matching Letters
MATERIALS: paper and pencil and any printed material one can mark up (a newspaper, a magazine, a piece of junk mail, etc.)
WHAT TO DO: Choose some printed material and put it on the table. Print a letter on the paper and ask the patient to mark every word that begins with that letter.

EXAMPLE:
If you choose an advertisement and the letter "b"
then he looks through the ad and marks every word beginning with "b."
Continue with other letters and printed material.
REMINDER: He can mark the letter by circling it, crossing it out, underlining it, or blackening it.
VARIATION: He can mark words containing the letter or words ending with the letter.
SIMPLIFYING THE ACTIVITY: Use a short paragraph.
EXPANDING THE ACTIVITY: Use several paragraphs.

_____ **ACTIVITY # 140:** Matching Letters
MATERIALS: paper and pencil and any printed material one can mark up (a newspaper, a magazine, a piece of junk mail, etc.)
WHAT TO DO: Choose some printed material and put it on the table. Print a combination of letters on the paper and ask the patient to mark every word that has that combination in it.

EXAMPLE:
If you choose a "letter to the editor" and the letter combination "st"
then he looks through the article and marks every word that has "st" in it.
If you choose an advertisement and the letter combination "ae"
then he looks though the ad and marks every word that has "ae" in it.
Continue with other letter combinations and printed material.

_____ **ACTIVITY # 141:** Matching Words
MATERIALS: paper and pen and any printed material one can mark up (a newspaper, a magazine, a piece of junk mail, etc.)
WHAT TO DO: Choose some printed material and put it on the table. Print a common word on the paper and ask the patient to mark that word every time he sees it.

EXAMPLE:
If you choose a paragraph from a magazine and print the word "is" on the paper
then he looks through the article and marks every "is" that he finds.
Continue with other words and articles.
REMINDER: He can mark the word by circling it, crossing it out, underlining it, or blackening it.
VARIATION: Print two words on the paper and ask him to find both words.

SIMPLIFYING THE ACTIVITY: Use a short paragraph.
EXPANDING THE ACTIVITY: Use several paragraphs.

_____ **ACTIVITY # 142:** Matching Words
MATERIALS: paper and pencil, felt-tip pen, and any printed material one can mark up (a newspaper, a magazine, a piece of junk mail, etc.)
WHAT TO DO: Choose five phrases from some printed material and write them down. Give the patient the list of phrases, a pencil, and the page of print, and ask him to look through the material and mark the phrases when he finds them.

EXAMPLE:
If you use an advertisement and you write the following phrases: "unconditional guarantee," "limited offer," "can't wait," "within ten days," and "intelligent person"
then he looks through the ad and marks those phrases when he finds them.
Continue with other phrases and printed material.
REMINDER: He can mark the phrases by circling them, crossing them out, underlining them, or blackening them.
SIMPLIFYING THE ACTIVITY: Write the phrases in the order in which they appear on the page.
EXPANDING THE ACTIVITY: You can write ten phrases instead of five. You can write more unusual phrases such as "in the," "of national," "are at," etc.

_____ **ACTIVITY # 143:** Recognizing Words
MATERIALS: paper, felt-tip pen, and pencil
WHAT TO DO: Print a sentence on the paper, but do not leave spaces between the words. Explain that you wrote it as if it were all one word. Give the patient the pencil and ask him to separate the words by putting lines between them.

EXAMPLE:
If you write "thebluecarpetneedscleaning"
then he makes lines like this: the/blue/carpet/needs/cleaning.
Continue with other sentences.
REMINDER: You can copy sentences from books, newspapers, or magazines.
EXPANDING THE ACTIVITY: Print several sentences together (without using punctuation) as if they were one sentence.

_____ **ACTIVITY # 144:** Recognizing Letters
MATERIALS: paper and felt-tip pen
WHAT TO DO: Print a capital letter on the paper, and ask the patient whether it is one of several different letters.

EXAMPLE:
If you print "G" on the paper and ask "is it the letter 'D'?"
then he says no.
If you ask "is it an 'R'?"
then he says no.
If you ask "is it a 'G'?"
then he says yes.
Continue by writing other letters.
REMINDER: Do not write the letters in alphabetical order. If he cannot speak, ask him to nod or shake his head.

_____ **ACTIVITY # 145:** Recognizing Letters
MATERIALS: paper and felt-tip pen
WHAT TO DO: Print any three capital letters in a row. Say one of the letters and ask the patient to point to it.

EXAMPLE:
If the letters "R," "D," and "Q" are printed on the paper and you say "point to 'Q' "
then he does it.
If you say "point to "R' "
then he does it.
Continue by printing three other letters.
EXPANDING THE ACTIVITY: Print the entire alphabet on the paper and ask him to point to any letter that you name.

_____ **ACTIVITY # 146:** Recognizing Letters
MATERIALS: paper and felt-tip pen
WHAT TO DO: Print a capital letter on the paper, and ask the patient to tell you what letter you printed.

EXAMPLE:
If you print "B"
then he says "B."
If you print "J"
then he says "J."
Continue by printing other letters.
REMINDER: Do not print the alphabet in order.

_____ **ACTIVITY # 147:** Recognizing Letters
MATERIALS: lined paper and pencil
WHAT TO DO: Say a letter of the alphabet, and ask the patient to write that letter on the paper.

EXAMPLE:
    If you say "R"
then he writes "R" on the paper.
    If you say "X"
then he writes "X" on the paper.
    Continue with other letters.
REMINDER: Do not say the letters in alphabetical order.

_____ **ACTIVITY # 148:** Recognizing Letters
MATERIALS: paper and felt-tip pen
WHAT TO DO: Print three words. Spell one of the words out loud, and ask the patient to point to the word you spelled.

EXAMPLE:
    Suppose you print these words: "table," "over," "horse."
    If you spell "o–v–e–r"
then he points to "over."
    If you spell "h–o–r–s–e"
then he points to "horse."
    Continue by writing three other words.
EXPANDING THE ACTIVITY: You can choose words which appear similar ("look," "lock," "lick") or which are long ("integrity," "integrate," "intellect").

_____ **ACTIVITY # 149:** Remembering Letters
MATERIALS: lined paper and pencil, felt-tip pen
WHAT TO DO: Print a word clearly on the paper, and tell the patient to look at it until he thinks he can write it from memory. When he is ready, cover the word, give him the pencil, and ask him to write it.

EXAMPLE:
    If you print "farm"
then he looks at it until he thinks he can remember it. He then writes it.
REMINDER: If he has trouble, uncover the word, and let him look at it a little longer. Ask him to try again.

_____ ACTIVITY # 150: Remembering the Alphabet
MATERIALS: lined paper and pencil
WHAT TO DO: Ask the patient to write the alphabet on the paper.
SIMPLIFYING THE ACTIVITY: Tell him what each letter is, then ask him to write it.

_____ ACTIVITY # 151: Spelling Words
MATERIALS: lined paper and pencil
WHAT TO DO: Spell a word out loud, slowly and clearly, and ask the patient to write the word on the paper as you spell it.

EXAMPLE:
    If you spell "t–o–e"
then he writes "toe."
    If you spell "f–e–a–r"
then he writes "fear."
    Continue with other words.
REMINDER: He can write each letter after you say it, or he can wait until you finish spelling the whole word before he starts writing.
SIMPLIFYING THE ACTIVITY: Use short words and say one letter at a time.

_____ ACTIVITY # 152: Spelling Words
MATERIALS: anything on which there is printing
WHAT TO DO: Point to a word, and ask the patient to spell it.

EXAMPLE:
    If you point to the word "country"
then he spells "c–o–u–n–t–r–y."
    Continue with other words.
VARIATION: Write a word for him to spell.

_____ ACTIVITY # 153: Alphabetizing
MATERIALS: letter tiles (see Appendix D)
WHAT TO DO: Place the tiles on the table so the patient can see them, and ask him to arrange the letters in alphabetical order.
REMINDER: Remove any duplicate letters before he begins.

_____ ACTIVITY # 154: Making Words
MATERIALS: letter tiles (see Appendix D)
WHAT TO DO: Using the tiles, form a word with a letter missing.

Place the tiles in front of the patient, leaving a space for the missing letter. Place three tiles (including the missing one) near the word. Have him select one of the letters to complete the word.

EXAMPLE:

Suppose you pick the letters T R A I N and two other letters such as O and E. You can arrange the letters like this: T R A N. Near this word put the other letters O I E. Then tell him to "pick one of the letters and make the word 'TRAIN.'"
He takes the letter I and puts it in the word so that it becomes TRAIN.

Continue by picking letters for other words.

REMINDER: You can leave out any letter in the word.

EXPANDING THE ACTIVITY: You can use longer words, or you can leave two blanks in a word and provide a choice of four letters from which to choose.

_____ **ACTIVITY # 155:** Making Words

MATERIALS: letter tiles (see Appendix D)

WHAT TO DO: Select letters and form a common word. Place the letters in front of the patient, but put them in the wrong order.

EXAMPLE:

Suppose the letters R A C D are on the table.

If you say "rearrange the letters so they spell CARD"
then he does it.

Suppose the letters W O P R E are on the table.

If you say "rearrange the letters so they spell POWER"
then he does it.

Continue to make different words with other letters.

SIMPLIFYING THE ACTIVITY: Show the patient the first letter of the word.

EXPANDING THE ACTIVITY: Use longer words.

_____ **ACTIVITY # 156:** Making Words

MATERIALS: letter tiles (see Appendix D)

WHAT TO DO: Select letters to spell a common word. Place the letters in front of the patient in the wrong order. Ask him to rearrange the letters to make a word but don't tell him what that word should be.

EXAMPLE:

If you put T U C S on the table and say "rearrange the letters to spell a word" *then he makes CUTS.*

If you put Y O N E M on the table and say "rearrange the letters to spell a word"
then he makes MONEY.

Continue by selecting more letters to form words.

VARIATION: Show the patient the first letter of the word.

SIMPLIFYING THE ACTIVITY: Give him hints about the meaning of the word he is to spell.

—————— **ACTIVITY # 157:** Making Words

MATERIALS: letter tiles (see Appendix D)

WHAT TO DO: Place ten different letters on the table, and ask the patient to make certain words from these letters.

EXAMPLE:

Suppose the letters D R J V S W E E O Y are on the table.

If you say "make the word 'yes' from the letters"
then he picks out the letters Y E S and forms the word.

If you say "make the word 'drove' from the letters"
then he picks out the letters D R O V E and forms the word.

Replace some or all of the letters and continue.

REMINDER: Make sure at least two vowels (A, E, I, O, U, Y) are among the ten letters.

—————— **ACTIVITY # 158:** Making Words

MATERIALS: letter tiles (see Appendix D)

WHAT TO DO: Place ten letters on the table. Ask the patient to take any of the letters and make a word of at least three letters.

EXAMPLE:

Suppose the letters P C B O R M N O A E are on the table.

If you say "pick three or more letters and make a word"
then he can make any of these: BROOM, BONE, BEAR, CAPE, MAN, CANOE, POOR, ROB, MANE, PROBE, NAME, etc.

Replace two of the letters with two different ones and continue.

VARIATION: After the patient makes one word, put the letter tiles back and ask him to make another. Continue having him make as many words as he can, using those same ten tiles.

SIMPLIFYING THE ACTIVITY: You can use six or eight tiles instead of ten, or you can suggest a word.

_____ ACTIVITY # 159: Identifying Letter Sounds
MATERIALS: none
WHAT TO DO: Pronounce a word, and ask the patient to tell you its
first letter.

EXAMPLE:
    If you say "what's the first letter in the word 'butter'?"
then he says "b."
    If you say "what letter does 'excellent' start with?"
then he says "e."
    Continue with other words.

_____ ACTIVITY # 160: Identifying Letter Sounds
MATERIALS: none
WHAT TO DO: Say a letter of the alphabet, and ask the patient to
say as many words as he can think of that begin with that letter.

EXAMPLE:
    If you say "tell me as many words as you can that begin with 'q' "
then he can say "quilt," "quiet," "quiz," "quickly," or any other word begin-
ning with "q."
    Continue with other letters.
VARIATION: You can ask him to write the words that he thinks of.
You can keep track of the number of words he gives for each letter
and compare this number when he does the activity at another time.
EXPANDING THE ACTIVITY: Ask him to think of words that end
with a certain letter.

_____ ACTIVITY # 161: Identifying Letter Sounds
MATERIALS: none
WHAT TO DO: Spell a letter combination, and ask the patient to say
as many words as he can with that combination in them.

EXAMPLE:
    If you say "name some words with 'st' in them"
then he can say "star," "story," "best," "last," "instant," "question," etc.
    Continue by saying other letter combinations.
VARIATION: Ask him to write words with these letters in them.
SIMPLIFYING THE ACTIVITY: Ask him to name one word that
has these letters in it.
EXPANDING THE ACTIVITY: Ask him to name as many words as
he can with these letters in them.

_____ **ACTIVITY # 162:** Recognizing Words
MATERIALS: paper and pencil
WHAT TO DO: Print three spellings of a word, only one of which is correct. Ask the patient to point to the correct spelling.

EXAMPLE:
If you write "palow," "pilo," and "pillow"
then he points to "pillow."
If you write "lamp," "lomp," and "linp"
then he points to "lamp."
Continue by printing other words.
SIMPLIFYING THE ACTIVITY: You can pronounce the correctly spelled word. You can make the incorrectly spelled words obviously wrong.
EXPANDING THE ACTIVITY: Make the spellings very similar.

_____ **ACTIVITY # 163:** Recognizing Words
MATERIALS: paper and felt-tip pen
WHAT TO DO: Print three different words, two of which are spelled correctly and one of which is spelled incorrectly. Ask the patient to point to the incorrectly spelled word.

EXAMPLE:
If you write "milc," "last," and "drag"
then he points to "milc."
If you write "sensible," "ocupay," and "umbrella"
then he points to "ocupay."
Continue by writing other words.
VARIATION: Print only one word that is spelled correctly and two that are not.
SIMPLIFYING THE ACTIVITY: Use familiar words which are easier to spell.
EXPANDING THE ACTIVITY: Use words which are not very common and may be hard to spell.

_____ **ACTIVITY # 164:** Spelling Words
MATERIALS: paper and pencil, felt-tip pen
WHAT TO DO: Print a word leaving out a letter. Leave a space for the missing letter. Give the patient the pencil and ask him to fill in the space with the correct letter.

EXAMPLE:
If you print B A N   N A
then he fills in the blank with an A to make the word BANANA.

If you print H O   E on the paper
then he can put one of several letters in the space to make a word such as
HOLE, HOME, HOPE, HOSE, or HONE.
Continue with other words.
SIMPLIFYING THE ACTIVITY: Say a word which he can make by
putting a letter in the space.
EXPANDING THE ACTIVITY: Leave more than one space in the
word so that he has to fill in more than one letter.

_____ **ACTIVITY # 165:** Recognizing Spelling
MATERIALS: none
WHAT TO DO: Spell a word out loud, slowly and clearly, and ask
the patient to tell you which word you have spelled.

EXAMPLE:
   If you say "l–e–a–f"
then he says "leaf."
   If you say "g–l–a–s–s"
then he says "glass."
   Continue with other words.
SIMPLIFYING THE ACTIVITY: You can use short, familiar words,
or you can spell the words, pausing between letters.
EXPANDING THE ACTIVITY: Use longer words.

_____ **ACTIVITY # 166:** Spelling Words
MATERIALS: none
WHAT TO DO: Say a word. Ask the patient to spell it.

EXAMPLE:
   If you say "spell the word 'car' "
then he does it.
   If you say "spell 'pencil' "
then he does it.
   Continue with other words.
SIMPLIFYING THE ACTIVITY: Use short, familiar words.
EXPANDING THE ACTIVITY: Use longer words.

_____ **ACTIVITY # 167:** Alphabetizing
MATERIALS: see checked items; paper, felt-tip pen
WHAT TO DO: Your clinician has checked some items to practice.
Choose one of them. Write something for the patient to look up in
one of the books. Ask him to find the item and show it to you.

———— Dictionary
———— Address book
———— Yellow Pages in a telephone book
———— White Pages in a telephone book
———— Index in a book

EXAMPLE:

Suppose you are using the index of a cookbook.
If you say "look up spaghetti"
then he finds it in the index and points to it.
If you say "find chocolate cake"
then he finds it and points to it.
Continue with other items.

SIMPLIFYING THE ACTIVITY: You can open the book to the page he will need. You can find the letter that begins the item he is looking for.

———— **ACTIVITY # 168:** Alphabetizing

MATERIALS: see checked items

WHAT TO DO: Your clinician has checked some items to practice. Choose one of them. Show the patient three things that are listed, and ask him to say them in alphabetical order.

———— Recipes
———— Titles of articles (from a table of contents)
———— Movie guides
———— TV shows
———— Table of contents in a book
———— Lists of words (three at a time)
———— Stack of books
———— Games
———— Ingredients in a product
———— Coupons

EXAMPLE:

Suppose you are using a movie guide in a newspaper, and the first three movies listed are *Ordinary People, Star Wars,* and *Sound of Music.*

If you say "put the first three movies in alphabetical order"
then he says "Ordinary People, Sound of Music, and Star Wars," in that order.
Continue with other things to alphabetize.

VARIATION: He can copy the items or point to them in the correct order instead of saying them out loud.

EXPANDING THE ACTIVITY: Ask him to put five items in alphabetical order instead of three.

_____ **ACTIVITY # 169:** Using Indexes
MATERIALS: a telephone book (Yellow and White Pages)
WHAT TO DO: Name some type of service and ask the patient to look it up in the phone book.

EXAMPLE:
If you say "look up florists"
then he finds florists in the Yellow Pages and shows you.
If you say "find a Chevrolet dealer"
then he can look up a specific dealer in the White Pages or find car dealers in the Yellow Pages and look for a Chevrolet dealer.
Continue with other items.
SIMPLIFYING THE ACTIVITY: Find the letter that begins the item he is looking for, or open the book to the page he will need.

_____ **ACTIVITY # 170:** Using Indexes
MATERIALS: a mail-order catalog
WHAT TO DO: Choose an item that is in the catalog. Give the patient the catalog and ask him to look for the item. When he finds it, ask him to tell you the page it is on, the brand name (if any), and the price of the item.

EXAMPLE:
If you say "look up glass fireplace doors"
then he finds them (using the index) and tells you the page number they are on, the brand name, and the cost.
Continue with other items.
REMINDER: You can choose a very general item (such as house paint) or a very specific one (such as a gallon of latex semi-gloss paint).
VARIATION: Ask him to write down the information or to fill out the order form in the catalog.
SIMPLIFYING THE ACTIVITY: Print the item which you want him to look up.
EXPANDING THE ACTIVITY: Ask him to write down the prices of the items as he finds them. When he has looked up several items, have him figure their cost, the tax, and the shipping charges.

Other Activities

Reading

Reading can take two different forms. The ability to recognize and read words out loud is one skill. The second and more important ability is to understand what words mean, that is, to understand the message that they convey. The person with aphasia may have difficulties in either area or both.

The majority of the activities in this section are for understanding what is read. For most of these activities the patient does not need to be able to speak. The last few activities deal with the ability to read out loud, so these do require him to speak. He does not, however, necessarily have to understand or be able to make sense out of what he is reading.

You will notice that a felt-tip pen is listed for Materials if a writing utensil is needed. This is because it makes a darker and bolder line than a regular pen and may be easier for the patient to see. However, a regular pen can be used as long as the patient finds your writing easy to read.

The following kinds of activities are done in this section on Reading:

Reading Words	Activities 171–77, 180, 185–86
Reading Phrases	Activities 178–79, 181–84, 187–93
Reading Directions	Activities 194–95, 200
Reading Sentences	Activities 196–99, 201–2
Reading Out Loud	Activities 203–6

Your speech-language pathologist will fill out this part.

Do _____ session(s) each day with the patient.

Do not spend any more than _____ minutes each session working.

_____ Correct any mistakes he makes.

_____ Do not correct his mistakes, but continue to the next question.

_____ Repeat the question if he makes a mistake.

_____ Keep track of any errors he makes.

_____ Do not keep track of his errors.

_____ Work on several activities at each working session.

_____ Work on only one activity during each working session.

Notes

_____ **ACTIVITY # 171:** Reading Words
MATERIALS: paper and felt-tip pen
WHAT TO DO: Print the name of an object on the paper, and ask the patient to show you how to use the object.

EXAMPLE:
    If you print "towel"
then he pretends he is holding a towel and drying himself.
    If you print "camera"
then he pretends he is holding a camera and taking a picture.
REMINDER: If he tries to describe the object, remind him that he is supposed to demonstrate its use without talking.

_____ **ACTIVITY # 172:** Reading Words
MATERIALS: paper and felt-tip pen, scissors, pictures of objects (see Appendix B)
WHAT TO DO: Print clearly the names of at least ten pictures that you will be using, at least one-half inch high, with enough room around them so that they can be cut out separately. Cut out the words and put them in front of you. Place one of the pictures on the table, and two of the words below the picture. Make sure one of the words

names the picture. Ask the patient to point to the word that names the picture.

EXAMPLE:

Suppose you put a picture of a banana on the table and the words "table" and "banana" below it.

If you ask "which word goes with the picture?"
then he points to "banana."

Replace the words and picture with different ones and continue.
REMINDER: Encourage him to say the words.
VARIATION: Use two pictures and one word so that he matches the word with the correct picture.
EXPANDING THE ACTIVITY: Place four words on the table instead of three and continue as before. If his answers remain correct, add a fifth word and continue until he has difficulty.

_____ **ACTIVITY # 173:** Reading Words
MATERIALS: paper and felt-tip pen, scissors
WHAT TO DO: Print clearly the names of about twenty things which can be found around the house, at least one-half inch high, with enough room around them so that they can be cut out separately. Cut out the words and place them in front of you. Give the patient one of the words, and ask him to take the name and place it on the object.

EXAMPLE:

If you give him the word "lamp"
then he goes to a lamp and puts the word on it.

If you give him the word "stove"
then he goes and puts the word on the stove.

Continue with other words.
REMINDER: Encourage him to say the words.
VARIATION: Tape the words to the appropriate items and ask him to read the names to you at different times throughout the day.

_____ **ACTIVITY # 174:** Reading Words
MATERIALS: paper and felt-tip pen
WHAT TO DO: Print three words across the top of a piece of paper. Say one of the words out loud, and ask the patient to point to the word you said.

EXAMPLE:

Suppose these words are on the paper: "duck," "cheese," "leaf."
If you say "point to 'cheese' "

then he does it.

If you say "which one is 'leaf'?"

then he points to it.

Continue with three different words.

VARIATION: You can cut words from newspapers or magazines and put three of them on the table. You can describe one of the words rather than naming it. For instance, you can ask him to point to the dairy product ("cheese"), the one with feathers ("duck"), or the one that comes from a tree ("leaf").

SIMPLIFYING THE ACTIVITY: Place two words on the paper instead of three.

EXPANDING THE ACTIVITY: Your clinician has checked some of the following types of words to use with this activity.

_____ Abstract words ("because," "while," "then")

_____ Words spelled similarly ("broad," "braid," "bread")

_____ Longer words ("electric," "discrimination," "development")

_____ Words with similar meanings ("big," "large," "huge")

_____ **ACTIVITY # 175:** Reading Words

MATERIALS: any books

WHAT TO DO: Place three books on the table. Say the title of one of them, and ask the patient to point to it.

EXAMPLE:

If you ask "which one is *War and Peace?*"

then he points to it.

If you ask "which one is *The Joy of Cooking?*"

then he points to it.

Replace any book he points to with a different one and continue.

VARIATION: Use magazines instead of books.

SIMPLIFYING THE ACTIVITY: Place two books on the table instead of three.

EXPANDING THE ACTIVITY: Place four books on the table instead of three and continue as before. If his answers remain correct, then add a fifth book. Add more books until he has difficulty.

_____ **ACTIVITY # 176:** Reading Words

MATERIALS: paper and felt-tip pen

WHAT TO DO: Print a list of familiar names on the paper. Say one of the names out loud, and ask the patient to point to the name you said.

EXAMPLE:

Suppose these names are on the paper: Frank (the patient's name), Louise (your name), John (his son's name), and Barb (his daughter's name).

If you ask "which one is John?"
then he points to it.

If you ask "which one is your daughter's name?"
then he points to it.

Continue by writing some other names in a list.

SIMPLIFYING THE ACTIVITY: Place two or three names at a time on the list.

EXPANDING THE ACTIVITY: You can use a longer list of names. You can use first and last names of neighbors, friends, relatives, and famous people.

_____ **ACTIVITY # 177:** Reading Words

MATERIALS: canceled checks

WHAT TO DO: Place three checks on the table. Name the person or business to whom the check was written, and ask the patient to point to that check.

EXAMPLE:

Suppose the checks are made out to the following: K-mart, Penney's, Visa.

If you ask "which one is made out to K-mart?"
then he points to the correct check.

Replace any check he points to with a different one and continue.

SIMPLIFYING THE ACTIVITY: Place two checks on the table instead of three.

EXPANDING THE ACTIVITY: Place four checks on the table instead of three and continue as before. If his answers remain correct, add a fifth check. Add more checks until he has difficulty.

_____ **ACTIVITY # 178:** Reading Phrases

MATERIALS: some mail (letters, junk mail, bills, etc.) Make sure there are return addresses in plain view either on the envelope or on a letterhead.

WHAT TO DO: Place three pieces of mail on the table. Identify one of the items, and ask the patient to point to that piece of mail.

EXAMPLE:

Suppose mail from Consumers Power, Burpee Seed Company, and Uncle Harry are on the table.

If you ask "which one is from the seed company?"
then he points to the envelope from the Burpee Seed Company.
If you ask "which one is from Uncle Harry?"
then he points to the correct one.
Replace any letter he points to with a different one and continue.
SIMPLIFYING THE ACTIVITY: Place two pieces of mail on the table instead of three.
EXPANDING THE ACTIVITY: Place four pieces of mail on the table instead of three and continue as before. If his answers remain correct, add a fifth piece of mail. Add more mail until he has difficulty.

_____ **ACTIVITY # 179:** Reading Phrases
MATERIALS: any printed material (a book, a magazine, mail, products with writing, packages with writing, etc.)
WHAT TO DO: Choose some printed material and place it on the table. Say a phrase that you can see somewhere on the item. Ask the patient to look for that phrase and point to it when he finds it.

EXAMPLE:
Suppose you use a table of contents in a magazine.
If you say "locate 'letters to the editor' "
then he looks and points to it.
If you say "show me the 'book review' "
then he looks and points to it.
Continue with other questions.
REMINDER: Do not point to the phrases in the order in which they appear on the page.
SIMPLIFYING THE ACTIVITY: Give him only a small amount of the printed material from which to choose. For instance, use one paragraph instead of three, half an index instead of a whole one, etc.
EXPANDING THE ACTIVITY: Give him an entire page of material from which to choose.

_____ **ACTIVITY # 180:** Reading Words
MATERIALS: paper and felt-tip pen
WHAT TO DO: Print three different words. Ask the patient a question that can be answered with one of the words, and tell him to point to the word that answers your question.

EXAMPLE:
Suppose you print the words "sweater," "laugh," "water."
If you ask "which one would you wear if you were chilly?"

then he points to "sweater."
    If you ask "which might you do if you just heard a joke?"
then he points to "laugh."
    Print three more words and continue.
REMINDER: Encourage him to say the word.
SIMPLIFYING THE ACTIVITY: Print two words instead of three.
EXPANDING THE ACTIVITY: Print four words instead of three
and continue as before. If his answers remain correct, add a fifth
word. Add more words until he has difficulty.

_____ **ACTIVITY # 181:** Reading Phrases
MATERIALS: crossword puzzles
WHAT TO DO: Place a crossword puzzle on the table. Read one of
the clues listed, and ask the patient to point to the clue that you read.

EXAMPLE:
    If you read "a city"
then he looks through the clues and points to it.
    If you read "in a state of wonder"
then he looks through the clues and points to it.
    Continue with other clues.
REMINDER: Do not say the clues in the order in which they are
listed.
SIMPLIFYING THE ACTIVITY: Have him look at only some of the
clues—just the across or down clues, the first five clues, etc.

_____ **ACTIVITY # 182:** Reading Phrases
MATERIALS: a menu, such as a carry-out menu. Some restaurants
will let you take away a menu if you ask for it. Sometimes parts of
menus will be printed in the newspaper.
WHAT TO DO: Place the menu on the table. Say the name of something that is listed, and ask the patient to look through the menu and
point to what you said.

EXAMPLE:
    If you say "find the chef's salad"
then he points to it when he finds it.
    If you say "point to the shrimp cocktail"
then he points to it when he finds it.
    Continue with other questions.
VARIATION: Ask him yes-or-no questions about the menu that he
can answer by nodding or shaking his head.
SIMPLIFYING THE ACTIVITY: Menus are usually divided into sec-

tions. Group the questions so that he can find the answers in one place, such as the section for appetizers, side dishes, desserts, etc.
EXPANDING THE ACTIVITY: If he is able, you can ask questions so that he has to read the answer out loud from the menu.

ACTIVITY # 183: Reading Phrases
MATERIALS: an index or table of contents
WHAT TO DO: Place the index on the table and open it to a page. Say the name of something that can be found on that page, and ask the patient to find it.

EXAMPLE:
If you say "find 'World War I' "
then he looks on the page and points to it.
If you say "find 'submarines' "
then he looks on the page and points to it.
Continue with other questions.
SIMPLIFYING THE ACTIVITY: Use only a part of the index or table of contents. Cover up the rest of the page.
EXPANDING THE ACTIVITY: You can start with the book closed and ask him to look up something. He can turn to the correct page in the book after he finds it in the index or the table of contents.

ACTIVITY # 184: Reading Phrases
MATERIALS: paper and felt-tip pen
WHAT TO DO: Print three phrases that we often say. Use one of the phrases in a sentence or story, and ask the patient to point to the appropriate phrase.

EXAMPLE:
Suppose you write the following phrases: "I'm hungry," "I'm fine," and "happy birthday."
If you ask "if you haven't had anything to eat all day what could you say?"
then he points to "I'm hungry."
If you ask "tomorrow Joe will be forty-five years old. What could you say to him?"
then he points to "happy birthday."
Write three more phrases and continue.
REMINDER: Encourage him to read the phrases out loud.
SIMPLIFYING THE ACTIVITY: Say one of the written phrases for him to point to.
EXPANDING THE ACTIVITY: Print four phrases instead of three

and continue as before. If his answers remain correct, add a fifth phrase. If his answers continue to be correct, let him look at all the phrases on the page while you explain a situation. He can choose his answer from the entire list.

_____ **ACTIVITY # 185:** Reading Words

MATERIALS: a map of a city, a state, or the United States

WHAT TO DO: Open the map and say the name of a place on the map. Ask the patient to find that place and point to it. Do not pick a place that is hard to find.

EXAMPLE:

Suppose a map of Michigan is on the table.

If you ask "where is Detroit?"

then he finds it and points to it.

If you ask "where is Grand Rapids?"

then he finds it and points to it.

Continue with other places on the map.

VARIATION: You can use a map showing street names so that he can look for a particular street. You can give him directions to follow to help him find the location you name.

SIMPLIFYING THE ACTIVITY: Use only part of the map and cover the rest.

_____ **ACTIVITY # 186:** Reading Words

MATERIALS: coupons

WHAT TO DO: Place three coupons on the table, and say the name of one of the products. Ask the patient to point to that coupon.

EXAMPLE:

Suppose these coupons are on the table: Windex, Bufferin, and Saran Wrap.

If you say "point to the one for Bufferin"

then he does it.

If you say "point to the one for Windex"

then he does it.

Replace any coupon he points to with a different one and continue.

SIMPLIFYING THE ACTIVITY: Place two coupons on the table instead of three.

EXPANDING THE ACTIVITY: Place four coupons on the table instead of three and continue as before. If his answers remain correct, add a fifth coupon. Add more coupons until he has difficulty.

_____ **ACTIVITY # 187:** Reading Phrases

MATERIALS: coupons

WHAT TO DO: Place three coupons on the table, and ask the patient a question that he can answer by pointing to one of them.

EXAMPLE:

If you ask "which one has 7 cents off?"
then he points to the correct answer.
If you ask "with which one can you get a free Coke?"
then he points to the correct coupon.
Continue with more questions, then change to different coupons.

SIMPLIFYING THE ACTIVITY: Place two coupons on the table instead of three.

EXPANDING THE ACTIVITY: Place four coupons on the table instead of three and continue as before. If his answers remain correct, add a fifth coupon. Add more coupons until he has difficulty.

_____ **ACTIVITY # 188:** Reading Phrases

MATERIALS: an advertising circular, a mail-order catalog, or a page of advertisements

WHAT TO DO: Open to a page with ads on it. Ask the patient a question about one of the ads. Tell him to look through the ads to find the answer and point to it.

EXAMPLE:

Suppose you are looking at some shoe ads.
If you ask "does this shoe come in brown?"
then he looks through the ads and answers.
If you ask "which shoe sells for $29.95?"
then he looks through the ads and answers.
Continue with other questions, then change ads.

SIMPLIFYING THE ACTIVITY: You can use two or three ads at a time, or you can use one that advertises different models of the same product.

_____ **ACTIVITY # 189:** Reading Phrases

MATERIALS: a TV guide or a program listing for one day

WHAT TO DO: Place the open guide on the table. Ask the patient a question about a TV show. Tell him to use the guide to find the answer.

EXAMPLE:

If you ask "what show is on at 8:30 A.M. on Channel 2?"
then he finds the answer and points to it.

If you ask "what time is a CBS special on tonight?"
then he finds the answer and points to it.
    Continue with other questions.
REMINDER: Encourage him to say the answer aloud.
EXPANDING THE ACTIVITY: Use a TV programming list for the week.

_____ **ACTIVITY # 190:** Reading Phrases
MATERIALS: movie listings or a movie guide
WHAT TO DO: Place the listing on the table. Pick out five theaters, cover the rest, or cut out the five you will be using. Ask the patient a question about a movie. Tell him to use the listing to find the answer.

EXAMPLE:
    If you ask "what is playing at the Somerset Theater?"
then he looks through the listing and points to the answer.
    If you ask "show me two theaters where *Wizard of Oz* is playing"
then he looks through the listing and points to the answer.
    If you ask "what time does the second show start at the Main Theater?"
then he points to the answer.
    Continue with other questions, then change ads.
REMINDER: Encourage him to say the answers aloud.
SIMPLIFYING THE ACTIVITY: Place listings for one or two movie theaters on the table.
EXPANDING THE ACTIVITY: Place more than five ads on the table or use the entire movie guide.

_____ **ACTIVITY # 191:** Reading Phrases
MATERIALS: recipes (from cards, newspapers, magazines, or cookbooks)
WHAT TO DO: Place a recipe on the table. It should have a separate list of ingredients that is easy to read. Ask the patient a question about one of the ingredients. Tell him to look through the recipe and point to the answer.

EXAMPLE:
    If you ask "how much flour do you put in the recipe?"
then he looks through the ingredients and points to the answer.
    If you ask "you use three tablespoons of what ingredient?"
then he looks through the ingredients and points to the answer.
    Continue with other questions, then change recipes.

REMINDER: Encourage him to say the answers aloud. Do not ask about the ingredients in the order in which they are listed.

EXPANDING THE ACTIVITY: Use the entire recipe including the directions on how to prepare the dish. Ask him questions that require looking through the entire recipe.

_____ **ACTIVITY # 192:** Reading Phrases

MATERIALS: a section of a newspaper or magazine with housing and real estate ads which includes a picture. Sometimes there are free brochures available in stores or banks showing houses for sale in the area.

WHAT TO DO: Choose four of the housing ads. If there are more than this on a page, either cut them out or cover the ones you are not using with blank paper. Ask the patient a question about one of the ads. Tell him to look through the ads to find the answer.

EXAMPLE:

If you ask "which house has four bedrooms?"
then he looks through the ads and points to the correct one.

If you ask "which house is selling for $98,000?"
then he points to the correct one.

If you point to a house and ask "does this one have a fireplace?"
then he looks through the ad and answers.

Continue with other questions, then change to different ads.

REMINDER: Encourage him to say the answer out loud.

VARIATION: Place four ads from the classified section (without pictures) on the table.

SIMPLIFYING THE ACTIVITY: Place two or three ads on the table instead of four.

EXPANDING THE ACTIVITY: Place five ads on the table instead of four and continue as before. If his answers remain correct, then add a sixth ad. If his answers are still correct, then use an entire page of housing ads with the pictures.

_____ **ACTIVITY # 193:** Reading Phrases

MATERIALS: the want ads or classified ads

WHAT TO DO: Open to a section of the ads. If there are more than five ads on the page, either cut them out or cover the ones you are not using with blank paper. Ask the patient a question about something in one of the ads, and tell him to look through the ads to find the answer.

EXAMPLE:
 Suppose you are looking at ads for cars.
 If you ask "how much is the 1978 Firebird selling for?"
then he looks through the ads and answers.
 If you ask "does the 1980 VW have an AM-FM radio?"
then he looks through the ads and answers.
 Continue with other questions, then change ads.
REMINDER: Encourage him to say the answer aloud.
SIMPLIFYING THE ACTIVITY: Place on the table two or three ads instead of five.
EXPANDING THE ACTIVITY: Place on the table a column of ads or all of the ads under a certain heading.

_____ **ACTIVITY # 194:** Reading Directions
MATERIALS: any medicines, prescriptions, or over-the-counter remedies
WHAT TO DO: Hand the patient a container. Ask him questions about how to use the medication, and tell him to look for the answers on the label.

EXAMPLE:
 Suppose he is holding a bottle of aspirin.
 If you ask "how many aspirin should an adult take?"
then he looks at the label and answers.
 If you ask "what are two reasons to take aspirin?"
then he looks at the label and answers.
 Continue with other questions, then change medications.
REMINDER: Encourage him to read the answer aloud from the label.
SIMPLIFYING THE ACTIVITY: Ask him yes-or-no questions that he can answer by nodding or shaking his head.

_____ **ACTIVITY # 195:** Reading Directions
MATERIALS: packages or cans of food
WHAT TO DO: Place a food item on the table. Show the patient the directions for preparing it, and ask him a question about how to make the food. Tell him to look through the directions, then answer.

EXAMPLE:
 Suppose he is holding a can of soup.
 If you ask "how many cans of water do you add to the soup?"
then he looks through the directions and answers.
 If you ask "how many servings does it make?"
then he looks through the directions and answers.

Continue with other questions, then change foods.
REMINDER: Encourage him to read the answer aloud.
SIMPLIFYING THE ACTIVITY: Ask the patient yes-or-no questions that he can answer by nodding or shaking his head.

——— **ACTIVITY # 196:** Reading Sentences
MATERIALS: the Yellow Pages of a telephone book
WHAT TO DO: Ask the patient a question that requires the use of the Yellow Pages to find the answer.

EXAMPLE:

If you say "show me the phone number of the Midas Muffler shop in town"
then he looks it up and points to the correct answer.
If you ask "how many Chevrolet dealers are listed?"
then he looks it up and counts the dealers.
If you ask "if you need your refrigerator fixed, who would you call?"
then he looks up the answer and shows you.
Continue with other questions.
REMINDER: Encourage him to read the answer out loud.
VARIATION: Suggest some specific places for him to look in the Yellow Pages.
SIMPLIFYING THE ACTIVITY: Open to one page and ask him questions that he can answer from that page.

——— **ACTIVITY # 197:** Reading Sentences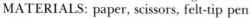
MATERIALS: paper, scissors, felt-tip pen
WHAT TO DO: Print in capital letters a five- or six-word sentence. Leave enough space around the words so that each can be cut out separately. Cut them out and put them in a pile, and ask the patient to rearrange them to make a complete sentence. (You can cut out more than one sentence at a time, but be sure to keep sentence parts together.)

EXAMPLE:

Suppose these words are on the table: CREAM COFFEE IN LIKE I MY
If you say "put the words in order to make a sentence"
then he rearranges them so that they read I LIKE CREAM IN MY COFFEE.
Continue by cutting out other sentences.
REMINDER: Encourage him to read the sentence aloud.

VARIATION: You can use sentences from magazines or newspapers. You can cut out headlines or titles of articles.
SIMPLIFYING THE ACTIVITY: Use short sentences.
EXPANDING THE ACTIVITY: Use longer sentences.

_____ **ACTIVITY # 198:** Reading Sentences ☆
MATERIALS: action pictures (see Appendix C), paper, felt-tip pen
WHAT TO DO: Choose a picture and put it on the table. Write a few words or a short sentence describing something in the picture, and ask the patient to point to the part of the picture that you described.

EXAMPLE:
If you write "the boat"
then he points to a boat in the picture.
If you write "the girl is holding the kitten"
then he points to that in the picture.
Continue by writing other things, then change pictures.
REMINDER: Encourage him to read aloud what you wrote.
SIMPLIFYING THE ACTIVITY: Write short descriptions as shown in the first example.
EXPANDING THE ACTIVITY: Write complete sentences as shown in the second example.

_____ **ACTIVITY # 199:** Reading Sentences ☆
MATERIALS: action pictures (see Appendix C), paper, felt-tip pen
WHAT TO DO: Place a picture on the table. Write a sentence about the picture, but make it incorrect in some way. Ask the patient to tell you what is wrong with the sentence.

EXAMPLE:
Suppose the picture has several people in it, including a man smoking a cigarette.
If you write "the man is smoking a pipe"
then he lets you know in some way that he knows that the word "pipe" is wrong. If he is able to speak he can tell you the man is smoking a cigarette, not a pipe. If he cannot, he can point to the word "pipe" and shake his head no, he can point to the man's cigarette, or he can gesture as if he were smoking a cigarette.
Continue with other sentences about the picture, then change pictures.

_____ ACTIVITY # 200: Reading Directions
MATERIALS: paper and felt-tip pen
WHAT TO DO: Write a direction for the patient to follow.

EXAMPLE:
If you write "make a fist"
then he does it.
If you write "put up two fingers"
then he does it.
If you write "make a square with a three inside it"
then he takes the pen and does it.
REMINDER: Encourage him to read the directions aloud.
SIMPLIFYING THE ACTIVITY: Write short directions.
EXPANDING THE ACTIVITY: Write more than one direction in the sentence, or write longer directions.

_____ ACTIVITY # 201: Reading Sentences
MATERIALS: any reading material which gives information. If the material is longer than a paragraph, then choose one paragraph.
WHAT TO DO: Ask the patient to read the item to himself. When he has finished reading, ask him some questions about what he read.
REMINDER: Encourage him to answer in sentences. If he cannot, ask him questions which he can answer in a few words.
SIMPLIFYING THE ACTIVITY: Ask him yes-or-no questions that he can answer by nodding or shaking his head.
EXPANDING THE ACTIVITY: Ask him to explain what he read in his own words. If he leaves out some important facts, ask him questions about them.

_____ ACTIVITY # 202: Reading Sentences
MATERIALS: any reading material
WHAT TO DO: Do the same as in Activity # 201. Make the reading materials longer, and provide more information.

EXAMPLE:
If you chose one paragraph from a magazine article in the previous activity, now use the whole article or three or four paragraphs.
REMINDER: Same as in Activity # 201.
SIMPLIFYING THE ACTIVITY: See Activity # 201.
EXPANDING THE ACTIVITY: See Activity # 201.

_____ **ACTIVITY # 203:** Reading Out Loud
MATERIALS: see checked examples
WHAT TO DO: This activity lets the patient practice reading out loud. Your clinician has checked some examples. Choose one of them and ask him to read the items out loud.

EXAMPLE:
_____ Words from a dictionary
_____ Names from an address book
_____ Names or services from a telephone book
_____ Word list from your clinician
_____ Names of products on coupons
_____ Words in an index
_____ Names of places on a map
REMINDER: If it is hard for him to say a word the first time he tries, say it for him. Ask him to repeat what you said.

_____ **ACTIVITY # 204:** Reading Out Loud
MATERIALS: see checked examples
WHAT TO DO: This activity lets the patient practice reading familiar material out loud. Your clinician has checked some examples. Choose one of them and ask him to read the item out loud.

EXAMPLE:
_____ Poems
_____ Riddles
_____ Jokes
_____ Limericks
_____ Organizations' pledges, creeds, rules, etc.
_____ Prayers, Bible verses
_____ Songs
_____ Months, days, holidays on a calendar
REMINDER: If it is hard for him to say a word or if he skips a word when he is reading, point to the word which is a problem. If he still has difficulty, say it for him, and ask him to repeat what you said.

_____ **ACTIVITY # 205:** Reading Out Loud
MATERIALS: see checked examples
WHAT TO DO: This activity lets the patient practice reading out loud. Your clinician has checked some of the following examples. Choose one of them, and ask him to read it out loud.

EXAMPLE:
_____ From newspapers: headlines, titles of features, section titles, names under photos
_____ From books: titles of chapters; names of characters, tables of contents
_____ From magazines: tables of contents, titles of articles
_____ From advertisements: the words in big type
_____ From cookbooks: lists of ingredients, names of recipes
_____ From the Yellow Pages: names of places, services, etc.
_____ From junk mail or letters: return addresses, information in big type
_____ From record albums: listings of songs, composers, singers, instruments
_____ From menus: foods, descriptions of dishes
_____ From food packages: lists of ingredients, directions
_____ From returned checks: name of payee
_____ From TV or radio program listings: names of shows, stars, descriptions
_____ From movie listings: names of movies, theaters, stars
_____ Postcards, greeting cards
_____ Labels, tags from clothing
_____ Crossword puzzle clues
_____ Want ads, classified ads
_____ Cartoons, comic strips
_____ Credit card names and information

REMINDER: If it is hard for him to say a word or if he skips a word when he is reading, point to the word for him to say. If he still has difficulty, say it for him, and ask him to repeat what you said.

_____ **ACTIVITY # 206:** Reading Out Loud
MATERIALS: a newspaper
WHAT TO DO: This activity lets the patient practice reading parts of a newspaper out loud. Some parts will be easier to read than others. Regular news articles will be the most difficult. Your clinician has checked some examples to practice. Choose one of them, and ask the patient to read it out loud. Some of the items listed may not be in your newspaper, but there may be others that are similar.

EXAMPLE:
_____ Weather reports
_____ Horoscopes
_____ Short summaries of news events
_____ Question and answer columns
_____ Short filler items about celebrities, unusual facts, etc.

_____ Schedules of events (entertainment calendars, meetings, clubs, etc.)
_____ Want ads, classified ads
_____ Sports scores
_____ Advice columns
_____ Captions under pictures
_____ Letters to the editor
_____ Other weekly or daily features

REMINDER: If it is hard for him to say a word or if he skips a word when he is reading, point to the word. If he still has difficulty, say the word for him, and ask him to repeat what you said.

EXPANDING THE ACTIVITY: You can ask him questions about what he has read. If he is able to speak well, you can ask him to talk about what he read.

Other Activities

Writing

The person with aphasia may have difficulty in expressing his thoughts in writing. This problem can be made worse if he cannot use his normal writing hand because of a weakness in it. The first few activities test the patient's ability to form letters and to copy them. It is suggested that you use a felt-tip pen for the model because it has a darker and bolder line and is easier to trace or copy. The patient is asked to use a pencil in case he needs to erase. (This may not be suitable for everyone, however, and your clinician may direct you to do something else.)

When someone is learning to write with a different hand, he usually has difficulty and begins by making large, awkward letters. You can make it easier for the patient if you make your own letters fairly large with extra space between them if he is to copy them. The patient may also find printing to be much easier than writing, or vice versa. Encourage him to use whichever approach seems more natural.

The following kinds of activities are done in this section on Writing:

Tracing Lines/Letters	Activities 207–8
Copying Shapes/Letters	Activities 209–11
Practicing His Signature	Activity 212
Copying Sentences/Information	Activities 213–15
Writing Words	Activities 216–20
Filling Out Forms	Activity 221
Taking Dictation	Activity 222
Writing Sentences	Activities 223–30, 232–34
Writing Questions	Activity 231

Your speech-language pathologist will fill out this part.

Do _____ session(s) each day with the patient.

Do not spend any more than _____ minutes each session working.

_____ Correct any mistakes he makes.

_____ Do not correct his mistakes, but continue to the next question.

_____ Repeat the question if he makes a mistake.

_____ Keep track of any errors he makes.

_____ Do not keep track of his errors.

_____ Work on several activities at each working session.

_____ Work on only one activity during each working session.

Notes

_____ **ACTIVITY # 207:** Tracing Lines

MATERIALS: felt-tip pen, paper, pencil

WHAT TO DO: Make several lines going in different directions with the felt-tip pen. Some of the lines should be straight, some slanted, and some curved. Give the pencil to the patient and ask him to trace over what you have drawn.

SIMPLIFYING THE ACTIVITY: You can draw one line, ask him to trace it, then draw another line, etc. You can draw three or four lines that look the same and have him practice with those. When he is able to trace them well, change the direction of the lines that you make.

EXPANDING THE ACTIVITY: Draw circles, squares, crosses, and other shapes as well as lines.

_____ **ACTIVITY # 208:** Tracing Letters

MATERIALS: felt-tip pen, lined paper, pencil

WHAT TO DO: Print a capital letter with the felt-tip pen. Give the pencil to the patient and ask him to trace over your letter. If he is able to do it, continue with other letters. Practice any letters that are difficult.

REMINDER: If he is using the hand that he does not usually write with, print your letters larger than usual. Use only capital letters and try all of the letters of the alphabet.

VARIATION: When he has traced the capital letters, you can print the lower-case letters. When he has traced those, then you can write them in cursive. You can also have him trace numbers.

EXPANDING THE ACTIVITY: Print a short word for him to trace.

_____ **ACTIVITY # 209:** Copying Shapes

MATERIALS: felt-tip pen, paper, pencil

WHAT TO DO: Make a design with felt-tip pen, using shapes and lines. Give the pencil to the patient and ask him to copy the design below it.

EXAMPLE:

If you draw a circle with a cross in it
then he copies it below your drawing.

If you draw two slanted lines going one way and two going another way
then he copies them.

Continue with other drawings.

EXPANDING THE ACTIVITY: Make your shapes and designs more complicated by using several figures and lines in each one.

_____ **ACTIVITY # 210:** Copying Letters

MATERIALS: felt-tip pen, paper, pencil

WHAT TO DO: Print a capital letter with the felt-tip pen. Give the patient the pencil and ask him to copy the letter below yours. If he is able to do it, continue with other letters. Practice any letters that are difficult.

REMINDER: If he is using the hand that he does not usually write with, print your letters larger than usual for him to copy. Use only capital letters and try all of the letters of the alphabet.

VARIATION: When he has copied the capital letters, you can print the lower-case letters. When he has copied those, then you can write them in cursive. You can also have him copy numbers.

EXPANDING THE ACTIVITY: Print a short word for him to copy below yours.

_____ **ACTIVITY # 211:** Copying the Alphabet

MATERIALS: felt-tip pen, paper, pencil

WHAT TO DO: Print the alphabet clearly with the pen. Leave space

between each letter, and about two inches between each line. Give the patient the pencil, and ask him to copy each letter below yours.
REMINDER: If he is using the hand that he does not usually write with, print your letters larger than usual.
VARIATION: Print a letter and ask him to look at it. Cover the letter, then ask him to print it.
EXPANDING THE ACTIVITY: You can print each letter in lower case. You can write each letter separately in cursive.

_____ ACTIVITY # 212: Practicing His Signature
MATERIALS: felt-tip pen, paper, pencil
WHAT TO DO: Your clinician has checked some instructions to practice. You will print (or write) the patient's name, and he will copy it.
_____ Print the letters for this activity.
_____ Write (in cursive) the letters for this activity.
_____ Ask him to copy each letter after you write it.
_____ Write his first name only.
_____ Write his last name only.
_____ Write his name and ask him to trace over your letters.
_____ Ask him to copy his entire name after you write it.
_____ Cover his name, and ask him to write it from memory.
REMINDER: The goal is for the patient to be able to write his signature when you ask him to do so.

_____ ACTIVITY # 213: Copying Information
MATERIALS: felt-tip pen, paper, pencil
WHAT TO DO: Your clinician has checked some examples to practice. Choose one of them. Print (or write, if the patient prefers) the information with the felt-tip pen. Give him the pencil, and ask him to copy what you wrote just below it.

EXAMPLE:
_____ His street address
_____ His city and/or state
_____ His entire address
_____ His telephone number
_____ Names of family members
_____ The date, day, and year
_____ Words describing the weather
EXPANDING THE ACTIVITY: Write one of the examples, then cover it with your hand. Ask him to write it from memory.

_____ **ACTIVITY # 214:** Copying Sentences
MATERIALS: felt-tip pen, paper, pencil
WHAT TO DO: Print (or write, if the patient prefers) a short sentence with the pen. Give the patient the pencil, and ask him to copy what you wrote below it.

EXAMPLE:
If you write "the car is red"
then he copies it.
If you write "the warm sun melted the snow"
then he copies it.
Continue with other sentences.

_____ **ACTIVITY # 215:** Copying Information
MATERIALS: see checked examples, paper, pencil
WHAT TO DO: Your clinician has checked some examples to practice. Choose one of them, decide what he is to copy, and ask him to copy what you show him. Do not ask him to copy too much during one session.

EXAMPLE:
_____ Dictionary: words, definitions of words
_____ White Pages of a telephone book: addresses and phone numbers
_____ Yellow Pages of a telephone book: listings under a certain heading
_____ Newspaper: headlines, horoscopes, ads, etc.
_____ Cookbook: lists of ingredients
_____ Menu: food listings, sample meals
_____ TV program listings: titles of shows, stars, etc.
_____ Radio guide: listings of songs, programs
_____ Record albums: listings of songs
_____ Letters: return addresses
_____ Want ads, classified ads
_____ Greeting card messages

_____ **ACTIVITY # 216:** Writing Words
MATERIALS: paper and pencil
WHAT TO DO: Say a short word that is easy to spell, and ask the patient to write the word on the paper.

EXAMPLE:
If you say "write the word 'cat' "
then he does it.

If you say "write the word 'line' "
then he does it.
Continue with other words.

_____ **ACTIVITY # 217:** Writing Words
MATERIALS: pictures of objects (see Appendix B), paper, pencil
WHAT TO DO: Place a picture on the table, and ask the patient to
write the name of the picture.

EXAMPLE:
If you show him a picture of a car and say "write the word for
this"
then he writes "car."
If you show him a picture of a shovel and say "write the word for
the picture"
then he writes "shovel."
Continue with other pictures.
REMINDER: If he misspells a word and asks for help, show him
which letters are correct and erase the others. Ask him to spell the
word again. If it is still wrong and he asks for help, spell the word
correctly while he writes it.

_____ **ACTIVITY # 218:** Writing Words
MATERIALS: paper and pencil
WHAT TO DO: Pick up or point to something that is in the room,
and ask the patient to write the name of the object.

EXAMPLE:
If you pick up a pillow and say "write the word for this"
then he writes "pillow."
If you point to a closet and say "write the word for this"
then he writes "closet."
Continue by pointing to other things.
REMINDER: If he misspells a word and asks for help, show him
which letters are correct and erase the others. Ask him to spell the
word again. If it is still wrong, and he asks for help, spell the word
correctly while he writes it.

_____ **ACTIVITY # 219:** Writing Words
MATERIALS: paper and pencil
WHAT TO DO: Ask the patient a question that he can answer in one
or two words, and tell him to write the answer on the paper.

EXAMPLE:
If you ask "what animal eats bananas?"
then he writes "monkey."
If you ask "what day is it?"
then he writes the day of the week.
Continue with other questions.
REMINDER: If he misspells a word and asks for help, show him which letters are correct and erase the others. Ask him to spell the word again. If it is still wrong and he asks for help, spell the word correctly while he writes it.

_____ **ACTIVITY # 220:** Writing Words
MATERIALS: paper and pencil
WHAT TO DO: Think of a category and tell the patient what it is. Ask him to write a word that will fit into the category.

EXAMPLE:
If you say "write the name of a country"
then he thinks of one and writes it.
If you say "write a kind of car"
then he thinks of one and writes it.
If you ask "what is something you should not eat if you are on a diet?"
then he thinks of something and writes it.
Continue with other categories.
REMINDER: If he misspells a word and asks for help, show him which letters are correct and erase the others. Ask him to spell the word again. If it is still wrong and he asks for help, spell the word correctly while he writes it.
EXPANDING THE ACTIVITY: Ask him to write two or three things in each category.

_____ **ACTIVITY # 221:** Filling Out Forms
MATERIALS: see checked examples, paper, pencil
WHAT TO DO: There are many types of forms that the patient can practice filling out. Your clinician has checked some to practice. Choose one for him to fill out.

EXAMPLE:
_____ Mail-order forms in catalogs
_____ Applications for credit cards, clubs, etc.
_____ Forms to enter contests
_____ Questionnaires, opinion or survey forms

_____ Subscription applications
_____ Change-of-address forms
_____ Forms for special offers, products, free merchandise
REMINDER: Sometimes the forms do not have enough room to fill in all the information. You can tell him to write the information on a piece of lined paper, or you can rewrite the questions on the paper.
VARIATION: Ask him to fill in an order form with whatever facts he chooses. He can include numbers, prices, or other information for the items.

_____ **ACTIVITY # 222:** Dictation
MATERIALS: paper and pencil
WHAT TO DO: Say a sentence out loud, and ask the patient to write the sentence exactly as you said it.

EXAMPLE:
If you say "it is cold outside"
then he writes it.
If you say "the glass fell on the floor"
then he writes it.
Continue with other sentences.
REMINDER: If he misspells a word and asks for help, show him which letters are correct and erase the others. Ask him to spell the word again. If it is still wrong and he asks for help, spell the word correctly while he writes it.
VARIATION: Read sentences from a book or magazine.
EXPANDING THE ACTIVITY: Use longer sentences.

_____ **ACTIVITY # 223:** Writing Sentences
MATERIALS: paper and pencil
WHAT TO DO: Say the first part of a sentence. Ask the patient to write it down and decide how to complete the sentence. Then tell him to write the rest of the sentence.

EXAMPLE:
If you say "the pan was . . ."
then he writes this part and finishes the sentence with an ending such as: *"dirty," "in the cupboard," "on the stove," etc.*
If you say "I wish I could . . ."
then he writes this part and finishes the sentence with an ending such as: "fly," *"go home," "win lots of money," etc.*
Continue with other sentences.
REMINDER: If he misspells a word and asks for help, show him

which letters are correct and erase the others. Ask him to spell the word again. If it is still wrong and he asks for help, spell the word correctly while he writes it.

SIMPLIFYING THE ACTIVITY: Use sentences in which he only needs to write one or two words to complete a thought.

—— **ACTIVITY # 224:** Writing Sentences
MATERIALS: paper and pencil
WHAT TO DO: Say a word, and ask the patient to write a sentence that contains that word.

EXAMPLE:

If you say "work"
then he can write "whistle while you work," "he was late for work," "I like to work with wood," etc.

If you say "dry"
then he can write "the well is dry," "dry your hands," "she put the dry clothes in the closet," etc.

Continue with other words.

REMINDER: If he misspells a word and asks for help, show him which letters are correct and erase the others. Ask him to spell the word again. If it is still wrong and he asks for help, spell the word correctly while he writes it.

EXPANDING THE ACTIVITY: Say two words and ask him to put both of them in one sentence.

—— **ACTIVITY # 225:** Writing Sentences
MATERIALS: photographs, paper, pencil
WHAT TO DO: Show the patient a photograph, and ask him to write about it.

EXAMPLE:

If you show him a personal family photograph
then he can write when, why and where it was taken, who is in it, etc.

If you show him a photograph from a book
then he can write what is in the photograph, what it reminds him of, why it might have been taken, etc.

Continue with other photographs.

REMINDER: Encourage him to write his answer in a complete sentence.

VARIATION: Ask him to write a caption for the photograph.

_____ **ACTIVITY # 226:** Writing Sentences
MATERIALS: action pictures (see Appendix C), paper, pencil
WHAT TO DO: Place a picture on the table, and ask the patient to write a sentence that says something about the picture.

EXAMPLE:
    If you point to a picture with a man in a boat
then he can write "the man is fishing from the boat," "the man is relaxing," "he hasn't caught any fish yet," etc.
    Continue with other pictures.
REMINDER: Encourage him to write his answer in complete sentences.
SIMPLIFYING THE ACTIVITY: Do not ask him to write a complete sentence.
EXPANDING THE ACTIVITY: Ask him to write a short story about the picture.

_____ **ACTIVITY # 227:** Writing Sentences
MATERIALS: paper and pencil
WHAT TO DO: Tell the patient to watch you. Pretend you are doing some kind of movement or action. Do not speak. Ask him to write about what you are doing.

EXAMPLE:
    If you pretend you are sneezing
then he writes "you are sneezing."
    If you stand up, go to a window, and rap on it
then he writes "you knocked on the window."
    Continue with other movements.
REMINDER: Encourage him to write his answer in a complete sentence.
EXPANDING THE ACTIVITY: Do more than one movement or action.

_____ **ACTIVITY # 228:** Writing Sentences
MATERIALS: paper and pencil
WHAT TO DO: Ask a question that the patient can answer in one sentence, and ask him to write down the answer to your question.

EXAMPLE:
    If you ask "why do you use an alarm clock?"
then he writes "I use an alarm clock to wake up," "I won't sleep late if I use an alarm clock," etc.

If you ask "where is Las Vegas?"
then he writes "Las Vegas is in Nevada."
 Continue with other questions.
REMINDER: Encourage him to write his answer in a complete sentence.

───── **ACTIVITY # 229:** Writing Sentences
MATERIALS: paper and pencil
WHAT TO DO: Tell the patient to look around the room, and ask him to write a description of something he sees.

EXAMPLE:
 Suppose there are flowers on a table.
He can write "the flowers are pretty," "there are different-colored flowers in a vase on the table," "I see pink, white, and yellow carnations in a vase," etc.
 Continue with other sentences.
REMINDER: Encourage him to write his answer in a complete sentence.

───── **ACTIVITY # 230:** Writing Sentences
MATERIALS: paper and pencil
WHAT TO DO: Ask the patient to write a sentence about something that happened recently.

EXAMPLE:
 The patient can write about several areas: personal things that happened to him, events in the news, things that have happened to others around him, things he has heard on the radio or television, etc.
VARIATION: Encourage him to keep a daily journal.
SIMPLIFYING THE ACTIVITY: Help the patient think of events that have happened, and ask him to write about one of them.

───── **ACTIVITY # 231:** Writing Questions
MATERIALS: paper and pencil
WHAT TO DO: Ask the patient to write a question for you to answer.

EXAMPLE:
 He can write "what time is it?" "what are we having for dinner?" "who was Jack Benny?" "where do pineapples grow?" etc.
 Continue with other questions.
VARIATION: You can use action pictures (see Appendix C) as a source for questions.

_____ **ACTIVITY # 232:** Writing Sentences
MATERIALS: paper and pencil
WHAT TO DO: Say a word, then ask the patient to write a sentence describing that word.

EXAMPLE:
    If you say "diamond"
then he can write "a diamond is expensive," "it is a precious gem," "a diamond is used in rings and other jewelry," etc.
    If you say "moist"
then he can write "moist means a little wet," "it means there's water in the air," "moist is like damp," "the cake is moist," etc.
    Continue with other words.

_____ **ACTIVITY # 233:** Writing Sentences
MATERIALS: pictures of objects (see Appendix B), paper, pencil
WHAT TO DO: Show the patient a picture, and ask him to write a complete description of what he sees.

EXAMPLE:
    Suppose the picture shows peanuts.
He can write a description such as "peanuts are small round nuts. They are hard and light brown. They are crunchy and roasted before we eat them. You can crush them to make peanut butter."
    Continue with other pictures.
REMINDER: Encourage him to write as many sentences as he wants in order to make a complete description.
SIMPLIFYING THE ACTIVITY: Ask him to write a sentence that tells how we use the object: for instance, "you eat peanuts" or "you use them to make peanut butter."

_____ **ACTIVITY # 234:** Writing Paragraphs
MATERIALS: see checked examples below, paper, pencil
WHAT TO DO: Your clinician has checked some examples to practice. Choose one of them, and ask the patient to write a paragraph or more about the topic.

EXAMPLE:
_____ Plot of a TV show or movie
_____ Plot of a book he has read
_____ Letter
_____ Answer to an editorial
_____ Opinion about an issue

_____ Step-by-step explanation of how to do something
_____ Explanation of an event in the news
_____ Story about a trip (one he has been on or one he would like to go on)
_____ Explanation of what he does during the day
_____ Report about an article or story
_____ Autobiography
_____ Explanation of aphasia and what it means to him
_____ Solving a problem (you pick the problem)

REMINDER: Encourage him to write more then one or two sentences.

Other Activities

Numbers

Sometimes the ability to count and to do arithmetic calculations is affected by aphasia. This section has activities for counting, recognizing numbers, saying and writing numbers, adding, subtracting, and solving problems.

Although the aphasic patient may not have trouble in using numbers, he may have difficulty in saying them. The reverse can also be true: he may not have difficulty saying them, but may have trouble in calculating or using them. Your clinician will indicate which activities are suited for the patient to practice.

The following kinds of activities are done in this section on Numbers:

Counting	Activities 235–37, 248
Recognizing Numbers	Activities 238–40, 242, 244, 247
Writing Numbers	Activities 241, 243, 245–46
Solving Problems	Activities 249–54
Using a Telephone	Activity 255
Using a Calendar	Activity 256
Telling Time	Activities 257–58
Recognizing Playing Cards	Activity 259

Your speech-language pathologist will fill out this part.

Do _____ session(s) each day with the patient.

Do not spend any more than _____ minutes each session working.

_____ Correct any mistakes he makes.

_____ Do not correct his mistakes, but continue to the next question.

_____ Repeat the question if he makes a mistake.

_____ Keep track of any errors he makes.

_____ Do not keep track of his errors.

_____ Work on several activities at each working session.

_____ Work on only one activity during each working session.

Notes

―――― **ACTIVITY # 235:** Counting

MATERIALS: none

WHAT TO DO: Ask the patient to hold up a certain number of fingers.

EXAMPLE:

If you say "hold up three fingers"
then he does it.

If you say "hold up eight fingers"
then he does it.

Continue with different numbers.

―――― **ACTIVITY # 236:** Counting

MATERIALS: none

WHAT TO DO: This activity helps the patient practice counting up to ten. Your clinician has checked some ways to do this. Choose one of them.

EXAMPLE:

―――― Put up a finger each time you say a number. He can watch you or do what you do.

_____ Say the numbers together slowly.

_____ Start by saying the numbers together, then fade your voice out when he is able to count alone.

_____ Use numbers or playing cards that are in order. As you put one down, have him say the number.

_____ Say "one" and "two" out loud while he says it with you. Then begin silently mouthing the words while he continues to count. If he has trouble, encourage him to watch your mouth for a clue.

_____ Print the figures 1 to 10 on paper. Point to the figure as you say it.

REMINDER: Count slowly and clearly.

EXPANDING THE ACTIVITY: When he is able to count from one to ten by himself, then repeat the procedure with numbers ten to twenty.

_____ **ACTIVITY # 237:** Counting

MATERIALS: none

WHAT TO DO: Hold up a certain number of fingers, and ask the patient to tell you how many fingers you are holding up.

EXAMPLE:

If you hold up seven fingers

then he says "seven."

If you hold up two fingers

then he says "two."

Continue with different numbers.

_____ **ACTIVITY # 238:** Recognizing Numbers

MATERIALS: felt-tip pen and paper

WHAT TO DO: Write the figures from 0 to 10 clearly with space between them. Say one of the numbers. Ask the patient to point to that number.

EXAMPLE:

If you ask "which one is eight?"

then he points to it.

If you ask "point to zero"

then he does it.

Continue by asking him other numbers.

EXPANDING THE ACTIVITY: Do the activity with the figures from 11 to 20. Then do the same thing with the figures from 1 to 20.

———— ACTIVITY # 239: Recognizing Numbers
MATERIALS: paper and pencil
WHAT TO DO: Give the patient the paper and pencil, and ask him to write the figures from 1 to 10.
SIMPLIFYING THE ACTIVITY: Tell him which number to write next.
EXPANDING THE ACTIVITY: You can ask him to write the figures from 11 to 20. You can turn over the paper and ask him to write the figures from 1 to 20.

———— ACTIVITY # 240: Recognizing Numbers
MATERIALS: paper and pencil
WHAT TO DO: Write the words for the numbers from one to ten down the side of the paper. Say one of the words, and ask the patient to point to that word.

EXAMPLE:
   If you say "point to six"
then he does it.
   Continue with other numbers.
EXPANDING THE ACTIVITY: You can write the words for the numbers from eleven to twenty. You can write the words for the numbers from one to twenty.

———— ACTIVITY # 241: Writing Numbers
MATERIALS: paper and pencil
WHAT TO DO: Give the patient the paper and pencil, and ask him to write the word for a number from one to ten.

EXAMPLE:
   If you say "write the word 'seven' "
then he does it.
   Continue with other numbers.
EXPANDING THE ACTIVITY: Have him write the word for any of the numbers from one to twenty.

———— ACTIVITY # 242: Recognizing Numbers
MATERIALS: paper and felt-tip pen
WHAT TO DO: Write any three figures on the paper with space between them. Say one of them out loud, and ask the patient to point to the number you said.

EXAMPLE:

Suppose you write 92, 46, and 54 on the paper.

If you say "point to 92"

then he does it.

If you say "which one is 46?"

then he points to it.

Write three more numbers and continue.

SIMPLIFYING THE ACTIVITY: Use the numbers from one to ten.

EXPANDING THE ACTIVITY: You can write down four figures on the paper instead of three. You can also make each one longer (563; 1,032), or you can make each of them similar in how they look and are said (2,042; 2,422; 4,242).

_____ **ACTIVITY # 243:** Writing Numbers

MATERIALS: paper and pencil

WHAT TO DO: Say a number, and ask the patient to write it down.

EXAMPLE:

If you say "twenty-four"

then he writes "24."

If you say "four hundred fifty-two"

then he writes "452."

Continue with other numbers.

SIMPLIFYING THE ACTIVITY: Say numbers under one hundred.

EXPANDING THE ACTIVITY: Say numbers over one hundred.

_____ **ACTIVITY # 244:** Recognizing Numbers

MATERIALS: felt–tip pen and paper

WHAT TO DO: Write the word for a number on the paper, then ask the patient to say the number out loud.

EXAMPLE:

If you write "seventy-five"

then he says it.

If you write "two hundred thirty-two"

then he says it.

Continue by writing other numbers.

SIMPLIFYING THE ACTIVITY: Write numbers under one hundred.

EXPANDING THE ACTIVITY: Write numbers over one hundred.

_____ **ACTIVITY # 245:** Writing Numbers

MATERIALS: pencil and paper

WHAT TO DO: Give the patient the pencil and paper, and ask him to write a certain group of figures.

EXAMPLE:

If you say "write the figures from 25 to 30"
then he writes 25, 26, 27, 28, 29, 30.
If you say "write the figures from 83 to 88"
then he writes 83, 84, 85, 86, 87, 88.
Continue by asking for other groups of figures.
SIMPLIFYING THE ACTIVITY: Use numbers under one hundred.
EXPANDING THE ACTIVITY: Use numbers over one hundred.

—————— **ACTIVITY # 246:** Writing Numbers
MATERIALS: pencil and paper
WHAT TO DO: Say a number, and ask the patient to write the word
for that number on the paper.

EXAMPLE:

If you say "sixty-three"
then he writes "sixty-three."
If you say "seventeen"
then he writes "seventeen."
Continue with other numbers.
SIMPLIFYING THE ACTIVITY: Say numbers under one hundred.
EXPANDING THE ACTIVITY: Say numbers over one hundred.

—————— **ACTIVITY # 247:** Recognizing Numbers
MATERIALS: see checked examples
WHAT TO DO: Your clinician has checked some examples to practice. Choose one of them, point to the numbers, and ask the patient to
say them out loud.

EXAMPLE:

—————— Phone numbers
—————— Sports scores
—————— Stock market numbers
—————— Temperatures from weather reports
—————— Prices of items in advertisements
—————— Page numbers in indexes or tables of contents
—————— Numbers on playing cards

—————— **ACTIVITY # 248:** Counting
MATERIALS: none
WHAT TO DO: Ask the patient to count to one hundred in a certain
way. Your clinician has checked some examples to practice. Choose
one of them.

EXAMPLE:
_____ Count by tens
_____ Count by fives
_____ Count by twos to fifty
_____ County by twentys
_____ Count by elevens
_____ Count backwards by one of the above
VARIATION: Use your own combination.

_____ **ACTIVITY # 249:** Solving Problems
MATERIALS: paper and pencil
WHAT TO DO: Write some simple arithmetic problems on paper, and ask the patient to solve them. Your clinician has checked the kind of problems to do (left column) and indicated how hard to make them (right column).

EXAMPLE:
_____ Adding   _____ Answers below 20
_____ Subtracting   _____ Answers below 50
_____ Multiplying   _____ Answers below 100
_____ Combinations of the above types

_____ **ACTIVITY # 250:** Solving Problems
MATERIALS: paper and pencil
WHAT TO DO: Write some arithmetic problems. Be sure to leave room for the patient to answer each problem. Your clinician has checked the type of problem to do.

EXAMPLE:
_____ Adding   _____ Answers below 50
_____ Subtracting   _____ Answers below 100
_____ Multiplying   _____ Answers below 1,000
_____ Dividing   _____ No limit to the answers
_____ Combinations of the above types

_____ **ACTIVITY # 251:** Solving Problems
MATERIALS: paper and pencil
WHAT TO DO: Tell the patient he is going to be solving math problems. Say a number, and ask him to write it. Say another number, and ask him to write it directly below the first one. After he writes them, ask him to solve the problem. Your clinician has checked some problems to do.

_____ Adding   _____ Answers below 20
_____ Subtracting   _____ Answers below 50
_____ Multiplying   _____ Answers below 100
_____ Dividing   _____ Answers below 1,000
_____ Combinations of the above types_____ No limit to the answers

EXAMPLE:

If you say "five hundred twenty-four"
then he writes 524.
If you say "one hundred thirty"
then he writes it directly below 524.
You can then say "add them together."
He does, and writes the answer "654."
Continue with other problems.

_____ **ACTIVITY # 252:** Solving Problems
MATERIALS: paper and pencil
WHAT TO DO: Say a simple arithmetic problem out loud, and ask the patient to answer the problem. Your clinician has checked the type of problem to use and its difficulty.

EXAMPLE:

If you ask "how much is three plus five?"
then he says "eight".
If you ask "how much is six times seven?"
then he says "forty-two."
Continue with other questions.

_____ Adding   _____ Answers below 20
_____ Subtracting   _____ Answers below 100
_____ Multiplying   _____ Answers below 1,000
_____ Dividing   _____ No limit to the answers
_____ Combinations of the above types

_____ **ACTIVITY # 253:** Solving Problems
MATERIALS: none
WHAT TO DO: Say several short arithmetic instructions in a row. When you finish, ask the patient to tell you the answer. Give him time to think of the answer before you add another step.

EXAMPLE:

If you say "start with ten (pause), add five to it (pause), and divide by three"
then he thinks and says "five."

SIMPLIFYING THE ACTIVITY: You can give problems with two parts. He can use paper and pencil to help him with the answer. You can ask him to tell you his answer after each step.

EXPANDING THE ACTIVITY: Say problems with three or more parts to them, such as "start with fifty, add seven, add nine, divide by six, multiply by four, and add one."

_____ **ACTIVITY # 254:** Solving Problems

MATERIALS: none

WHAT TO DO: Make up some math story problems, and ask the patient to tell you the answers.

EXAMPLE:

   If you ask "how many pills would you take in one day if you had to take three pills every six hours?"

then he says "twelve pills."

   If you ask "there are going to be four couples at a party. Each person will have four drinks. How many drinks will be needed?"

then he says "thirty-two drinks."

VARIATION: Your clinician has checked some examples to practice:

_____ Changing to inches, feet, yards

_____ Changing to ounces, pounds

_____ Changing to pints, quarts, gallons

_____ Doubling or halving ingredients in a recipe

_____ Figuring miles per gallon of gas

_____ Figuring percentages

_____ Figuring taxes on purchases

_____ Figuring meters, liters, grams, etc.

_____ Figuring distances between places (use a map)

_____ Figuring length of time to travel, to cook something, etc.

_____ Figuring calories in a meal or day (use calorie chart)

EXPANDING THE ACTIVITY: Make the problems longer and more difficult.

_____ **ACTIVITY # 255:** Using a Telephone

MATERIALS: a telephone

WHAT TO DO: This activity is done to practice dialing numbers. Leave the receiver on the hook. Think of a phone number. Say one number at a time. After you say each number, ask the patient to dial it. If he does it correctly, go on to the next number. Continue with other numbers.

REMINDER: He will be pushing buttons if you have a push-button phone.

VARIATION: You can write the number for him to dial. You can point to a number in the phone book for him to dial.

EXPANDING THE ACTIVITY: You can say the phone number that he will dial in groups of numbers or all at once. You can tell him to dial a number that he knows by heart.

_____ **ACTIVITY # 256:** Using a Calendar

MATERIALS: a calendar that is easy to read

WHAT TO DO: Your clinician has checked some examples to practice. Choose one of them, and follow the instructions.

EXAMPLE:

_____ Point to a date and ask him to read it (include the day, number, and month).

_____ Say a date and ask him to point to it.

_____ Ask him to say the days of the week.

_____ Ask him to say the months of the year.

_____ Ask him to tell you the number of days in each month.

_____ Name a certain date and ask him to point to it. For instance, if you say "what date is two days before the thirtieth?" *then he points to 28.*

_____ **ACTIVITY # 257:** Telling Time

MATERIALS: paper and felt-tip pen, two flat toothpicks or something similar

WHAT TO DO: Draw a large clock face on a sheet of paper. Use the toothpicks as the "hands" of the clock. Place the toothpicks so that they show a time on the clock, and ask the patient to tell you what time it is.

VARIATION: Give him the toothpicks, and say a time. Ask him to place the toothpicks on the clock so that they show that time. You can ask him to write down the time the clock shows.

SIMPLIFYING THE ACTIVITY: Put the toothpicks on only the hour or half hour.

_____ **ACTIVITY # 258:** Telling Time

MATERIALS: a clock

WHAT TO DO: At several times during the day, ask the patient what time it is. Have him look at a clock or watch to tell you.

SIMPLIFYING THE ACTIVITY: Ask him if it is a certain time of the day so that he can answer yes or no.

_____ **ACTIVITY # 259:** Recognizing Playing Cards

MATERIALS: one or two decks of playing cards

WHAT TO DO: Your clinician has checked some examples to practice. Choose one of them, and follow the instructions.

EXAMPLE:

_____ Separate one suit from the deck. Shuffle the cards and spread them on the table face up. Name one of the cards, and ask the patient to point to it.

_____ Shuffle one deck. Turn over the first card, and ask him to name its number and suit.

_____Usetwo decks and shuffle each one separately. Give him one deck and keep the other. Turn over the first card in your deck, and ask him to find that card in his deck.

_____ Use two decks. Shuffle one deck and separate the other into suits. Put the four piles in front of him. Turn over the first card in your shuffled deck and show it to him. Ask him to look in the correct pile to find it.

_____ Give him a deck of cards. Ask him to arrange it into suits, then arrange each suit in order from ace to king.

Other Activities

Money

This section concentrates on the uses of money in different situations. Sometimes the aphasic person can identify or count money, but cannot figure out how to use it properly for a purchase. Sometimes the aphasic person can recognize types of money, but cannot count it or add it.

These activities concentrate on money skills. Your clinician has checked some of these activities for the patient to do.

The following kinds of activities are done in this section on Money:

Recognizing Coins/Bills	Activities 260–61
Counting Coins/Bills	Activities 262–66
Writing Amounts	Activity 268
Recognizing Amounts	Activities 267, 269–71
Solving Problems	Activities 272–73

Your speech-language pathologist will fill out this part.

Do _____ session(s) each day with the patient.

Do not spend any more than _____ minutes each session working.

_____ Correct any mistakes he makes.

_____ Do not correct his mistakes, but continue to the next question.

_____ Repeat the question if he makes a mistake.

_____ Keep track of any errors he makes.

_____ Do not keep track of his errors.

_____ Work on several activities at each working session.

_____ Work on only one activity during each working session.

Notes

_____ **ACTIVITY # 260:** Recognizing Money
MATERIALS: coins and bills. Try to have more than one of each kind up to a twenty-dollar bill.
WHAT TO DO: Place a coin or bill in front of the patient, and ask him to tell you what it is.

EXAMPLE:
    If you give him a quarter and ask "what is this?"
    then he says "a quarter."
    Continue with other questions.
VARIATION: Also ask "how much is it worth?"

_____ **ACTIVITY # 261:** Recognizing Money
MATERIALS: coins and bills. Try to have more than one of each kind up to a twenty-dollar bill.
WHAT TO DO: Place the money in front of the patient. Say the name of one piece, and ask him to point to the one you named.

EXAMPLE:
    If you say "where is the five-dollar bill?"
    then he points to it.
    If you say "point to the quarter"
    then he does it.
    Continue with other questions.

_____ **ACTIVITY # 262:** Counting Money
MATERIALS: a lot of loose change
WHAT TO DO: Place all of the money in front of the patient, and ask him to give you a certain combination of coins.

EXAMPLE:
    If you say "give me two nickels and four pennies"
    then he finds them and gives them to you.
    Put all the money back together and continue.
    If you say "find three quarters, a dime, and two pennies"
    then he does it.
    Put all the money back together and continue.

_____ **ACTIVITY # 263:** Counting Money
MATERIALS: a lot of loose change
WHAT TO DO: Place the money in front of the patient, and ask him to remove a certain amount.

EXAMPLE:

If you say "show me thirty-two cents"

then he might give you a quarter, a nickel, and two pennies (or other coins equal to thirty-two cents).

If you say "give me a dollar and eighty-seven cents"

then he might give you six quarters, three dimes, and seven pennies.

Put all the money back together and continue.

REMINDER: Do not ask him for more money than is on the table.

EXPANDING THE ACTIVITY: Use bills and change and ask him for larger amounts.

_____ **ACTIVITY # 264:** Counting Money

MATERIALS: paper and pencil, a lot of loose change

WHAT TO DO: Place the change in front of the patient. Write down a sum of money, show him the amount you wrote, and ask him to remove that amount from the pile.

EXAMPLE:

If you write $.63

then he might give you two quarters, one dime, and three pennies (or other coins equal to $.63).

Put all the money together and continue.

If you write $2.41

then he might give you six quarters, one-half dollar, three dimes, two nickels, and one penny (or other coins equal to $2.41).

Put all the money back together and continue.

REMINDER: Do not write a sum greater than the amount of money on the table.

EXPANDING THE ACTIVITY: Use bills and change and write larger amounts.

_____ **ACTIVITY # 265:** Counting Money

MATERIALS: a lot of loose change, some bills

WHAT TO DO: Place the money in front of the patient, and tell him to remove different amounts of money as you say them. After that, ask him to tell you the total amount of money that he has removed from the pile.

EXAMPLE:

If you say "remove fifty-two cents"

then he does it.

Then ask him to "remove twenty-seven cents"

and he does this.

You then can ask "how much money is that all together?"
and he adds them and says "seventy-nine cents."

Put all the money back together and continue.

REMINDER: Do not ask him for more money than is on the table.

EXPANDING THE ACTIVITY: Ask him to remove three amounts of money instead of two.

_____ **ACTIVITY # 266:** Counting Money

MATERIALS: a lot of loose change

WHAT TO DO: Place several of the coins in front of the patient. Ask him to add the coins and tell you the total amount.

EXAMPLE:

If you place two quarters, three dimes, and one penny in front of him and ask "how much is that?"
then he adds them and says "eighty-one cents."

If you place two nickels, a half-dollar, three quarters, and a dime in front of him and ask "how much is that?"
then he adds them and says "one dollar and forty-five cents."

Put the money back together, remove several coins, add some others, and continue.

EXPANDING THE ACTIVITY: Give him bills and change and ask him for larger amounts of money.

_____ **ACTIVITY # 267:** Recognizing Amounts of Money

MATERIALS: canceled checks

WHAT TO DO: Place three checks on the table. Say the amount of money that is on one of the checks, and ask the patient to point to the check that is written for that amount.

EXAMPLE:

Suppose checks for $62.00, $47.53, and $17.50 are on the table.

If you say "point to the check for forty-seven dollars and fifty-three cents"
then he does it.

If you say "which one is for sixty-two dollars?"
then he points to it.

Replace any check he points to with a different one and continue.

_____ **ACTIVITY # 268:** Writing Amounts of Money

MATERIALS: paper and pencil

WHAT TO DO: Say an amount of money, and ask the patient to write that amount as if he were writing a check.

EXAMPLE:
If you say "twelve dollars and ten cents"
then he writes it.
Continue with other amounts.
REMINDER: There are several ways to write amounts of money on a check. Tell him to write the amount as he is used to doing it.
VARIATION: Practice with some old blank checks.

_____ **ACTIVITY # 269:** Recognizing Amounts of Money
MATERIALS: a newspaper or advertising circular
WHAT TO DO: Place a page with easy-to-read prices on the table. Point to any one of the items on the page, and ask the patient to tell you how much it costs.

EXAMPLE:
If you point to an ad for a color TV and ask "how much is it?"
then he tells you the price.
Continue with other items.

_____ **ACTIVITY # 270:** Recognizing Amounts of Money
MATERIALS: a newspaper or advertising circular
WHAT TO DO: Place a page with easy-to-read prices on the table. Say the price of one of the items on the page, and ask the patient to find the item selling for that price and point to it.

EXAMPLE:
Suppose the ad is for lawn mowers. If you ask "which one costs $234?"
then he finds it and points to it.
Continue with other questions.
VARIATION: If you find several items selling for the same price, ask him to point to all of these.

_____ **ACTIVITY # 271:** Recognizing Amounts of Money
MATERIALS: pictures of objects (see Appendix B)
WHAT TO DO: Place two pictures in front of the patient, and ask him to point to the item that is the most expensive.

EXAMPLE:
Suppose pictures of a bar of soap and a rake are on the table.
If you ask "which one is more expensive?"
then he points to the rake.
Replace the picture he named with a different one and continue.

VARIATION: Ask him to name the least expensive one.
SIMPLIFYING THE ACTIVITY: Use objects which are very different in price.
EXPANDING THE ACTIVITY: You can use three pictures instead of two. You can ask him to put the pictures in order from least to most expensive.

_____ **ACTIVITY # 272:** Solving Problems
MATERIALS: paper and pencil, food ads that give prices for the items. These can be ads from a newspaper, ad circulars from the mail or from a grocery store, etc.
WHAT TO DO: Choose a page of ads. Write down an imaginary shopping list of five items shown in the ads. Ask the patient to look through the ads and write down the price of each item as he finds it. After he finishes, ask him to add up the prices and tell you the total amount of money needed to buy those items.
SIMPLIFYING THE ACTIVITY: Write down two items instead of five.
EXPANDING THE ACTIVITY: You can say more than one of each food item. For instance, you can order two pounds of hamburger instead of one. You can ask him to include tax and tip in his total.

_____ **ACTIVITY # 273:** Solving Problems
MATERIALS: advertisements of items which also give the prices. These can be ads from a newspaper, ad circulars, brochures, etc.
WHAT TO DO: Write an amount of money on the paper, and ask the patient to look through the ads to find some things to buy. The amount of money that you write down is how much he can "spend." Tell him to choose items that, when added together, do not exceed the amount written down. Tell him to try to come as close as he can to that amount without going over it.

EXAMPLE:
Suppose there is an ad from an appliance store, and you have written "$50.00."
He can "buy" a hair dryer for $16.95 and a toaster for $31.99. Then his total is $48.94.
Continue with other amounts.
REMINDER: You can use any amount of money.
VARIATION: You can use a gift or mail order catalog instead of the ads.

Other Activities

GAMES AND OTHER PASTIMES

Introduction

Relearning speech and language skills need not all be hard work. Many things are now on the market that provide an excellent addition to aphasia treatment, including games, word puzzles, and electronic devices which can be used by both patient and family members to encourage communication.

The games listed in this section will require that you and the patient spend time on speech and language activities. Practicing these skills in a relaxed, enjoyable, family-oriented setting is very helpful to success.

A variety of games is listed to help aphasic patients develop communication skills in a successful manner. These games are challenging, fun, and often helpful in bringing the family together.

M. R.

How To Use Games and Other Pastimes

The listing that follows represents the author's choice of games and activities which have been screened by aphasic patients and found to be suitable. However, a patient's individual preferences and communicative difficulties must be taken into consideration before trying a game.

This section is divided into six parts. Most games in the first five sections require two or more players. The last section suggests things for the patient to do by himself. The games within the headings are listed in order of easiest to hardest. A description of each game is included along with the name of the company that makes it. An idea of the skills that the patient will need in order to play the game is also given.

There are other good games on the market which you can check, including children's games. Although an item may be intended for young children, it may be fun for adults, even educational and challenging for the patient. Before you use a new game, try one that is familiar to the patient. An important point to consider is that you may be able to change the rules in a number of games to make it easier for the patient to participate. Any game, in the end, is really only a suggestion: you can change it to suit your needs in any way you want. If you have any doubts as to what your family member should try, ask your speech-language pathologist for advice.

The games listed appear to be those most easily available across the country and most appealing to adults. This list needs to be kept current because games go on and off the market frequently (see the Suggestion Form at the end of this book). You may find these games in department stores, large drug or chain stores, toy stores, or even in stores that have only a small selection of games. The games you can buy will often depend on what is popular in your area, and so your selection may often change.

Matching Games

The patient need not be able to talk nor need he have any other special skills. He will have to be able to match patterns, shapes, or pictures to each other to play these games. Their rules can all be changed to allow the patient to use them by himself.

Lotto. In this beginner's game, the patient matches pictures that look the same. There are several versions available: the Milton Bradley Company has some which are more difficult to play and which require the matching of related items. 1 or more players.

Dominoes. This is a basic matching game in which one recognizes and matches patterns on the dominoes. Many companies sell domino sets. 1 or more players.

Tri-Ominos, Quad-Ominos by Pressman. Played like dominoes, Tri-Ominos is similar except that the pieces have three sides with numbers printed on them. Quad-Ominos has four sides. 1 or more players.

Picture Tri-Ominos by Pressman. Played like dominoes, the game pieces look like Tri-Ominos except that they have colored pictures with numbers on them. 1 or more players.

Stack-Ominos by Pressman. This is similar to, but more complicated than, dominoes because here the dominoes are stacked on top of one another in certain ways instead of side by side. 1 or more players.

Perfection and **Superfection** by Lakeside. Perfection involves matching shapes; Superfection uses three-dimensional shapes that fit together. The object is to fit the shapes where they belong within a time limit. 1 or more players.

Trac 4 by Lakeside. This matching game is more difficult because of the way the patterns are arranged. The object is to copy a pattern using cubes and to pick that pattern from a "revolving tower." This can be changed to make it easier for the patient. 1 or more players.

Memory Card Matching Game by Milton Bradley. This game is good practice in remembering what you see and where you see it. The game uses pictures, and the object is to find two that are alike. 1 or more players.

Concentration by Milton Bradley. This game employs the same idea as Memory Card Matching Game (remembering where you see pictures) but has some variations to make it more difficult. 1 or more players.

Games with Numbers and Dice

The patient need not be able to talk to play these games. He does have to be able to recognize and use numbers or throw dice and move markers.

Bingo. In this familiar game, the patient has to recognize numbers from 1 to 100. There are many versions that you can buy. 2 or more players.

Racko by Cadaco. The patient needs to be able to recognize the numbers from 1 to 100 and to arrange them from lowest to highest. The object of the game is to pick up and then get rid of cards until you have ten cards that go from low to high. 2–4 players.

Payday by Parker Brothers. The patient needs to be able to count and use money. This game board has a "month" through which players move and pay bills as they go along, based on typical monthly bills. There is "mail" that will have to be read to those patients who cannot read. 2–4 players.

Aggravation by Lakeside, **Parcheesi** by Selchow and Righter, **Sorry** by Parker Brothers. These are all board games with slight differences in rules. The patient needs to be able to count dice and move a marker. 2–4 players.

Yahtzee by Milton Bradley. The patient needs to be able to recognize the numbers on the dice, group them, and add them. The object is to throw five dice and arrange them to fit into certain categories on a score sheet. The play and decisions are slightly more complicated than in previous games. If the patient cannot keep his own score, someone can do it for him. There are several versions of Yahtzee as well as other very similar games put out by different companies. They all follow the same general idea, and the rolls may be for poker hands, bowling scores, etc. 1 or more players.

Backgammon. Several companies sell this game. The patient needs to be able to group the dice in order to move markers. The object is for each player to get his markers off the board before his opponent does. Luck and logic play a part in this game. 2 players.

Can't Stop by Parker Brothers. The patient needs to be able to group the dice in order to move markers. Luck and logic are involved. The patient may have some difficulty remembering the rules at first. 2–4 players.

Easy Money by Milton Bradley, **Go for Broke** by Selchow and Righter, **Life** by Milton Bradley, **Monopoly** by Parker Brothers. These board games are very much alike. Probably the most familiar one is Monopoly. Most of the difficulty for an aphasic person will probably be in learning the rules and using the money. Reading, talking, and strategy are not necessary in order to play. 2 or more players.

Strategy Games

The patient need not be able to talk to play these games, which are listed together because there is a certain amount of thinking, planning, and logic involved in playing them. The actual playing of these games is easy to learn. There are many more difficult strategy games on the market if you find the ones in this listing too easy. However, you will need to check the directions of each one to see if you think the patient can play it.

Tic Tac Toe. You can either buy this standard game or use pencil and paper. 2 players.

Tic Tac Toe Times 10 by Selchow and Righter. This game is listed separately because it is more detailed than a regular Tic Tac Toe game. 2 players.

Score 4 by Lakeside. This is a three-dimensional version of Tic Tac Toe. 2 players.

Checkers. Almost everyone has played this game at one time or another. Once a patient recalls the rules, he usually does not have too much difficulty playing it. 2 players.

Chinese Checkers. Several companies sell this game, in which you jump your markers over other markers in order to get across the board first. 2–6 players.

Take 5 by Gabriel. The object is to get five markers in a row before your opponent does. 2 players.

Connect 4 by Milton Bradley. The object is to get four checkers in a row by sliding them onto a vertical board. 2 players.

Mastermind by Invicta. Thinking, logic, and reasoning skills are important in this game. One player chooses a "secret" pattern of four colored pegs and the other player tries to guess the pattern. The game can be made easier for the aphasic patient by using fewer pegs or colors. 2 players.

Spelling and Word Games

The patient need not be able to talk to play these games, but he must have some ability to spell and, especially, to recognize and pick out words from a number of scrambled letters. Three games require writing words, but the rules can be changed for the patient who is unable to write.

Scrabble Crossword Dominoes by Selchow and Righter. These are domino shapes with letters on them. The object is to put them together to spell three- or four-letter words. 1 or more players.

Ad Lib by Milton Bradley, **Perquackey** by Lakeside, **Scrabble Crossword Cubes Game** by Selchow and Righter, **Spill and Spell** by Parker Brothers. The patient needs to be able to recognize words in scrambled form and to spell them out. The games are all played the same way and consist of dice with letters on them. 1 or more players.

Scrabble, Scrabble for Juniors by Selchow and Righter. In this popular game, the patient needs to be able to recognize words in scrambled form and be able to spell them. 2–4 players.

Boggle, Big Boggle by Parker Brothers. The patient needs to be able to guess a word from letter clues. In addition, he also needs to think of and write a word, but someone can write for him if necessary. 2–4 players.

Scrabble Sentence Cubes by Selchow and Righter. For this game the patient has to be able to read, not spell, words. The object is to form sentences from dice with words on them. 1 or more players.

Probe by Parker Brothers. The patient needs to be able to guess a word from letter clues. In addition, he needs to think of and spell a word with alphabet cards. 2–4 players.

Facts in Five by Avalon Hill. The object is to write words in a given subject area beginning with a certain letter of the alphabet. The game can be changed so that the patient who cannot read or write can still play if others read to him and he says his answers. 1 or more players.

Password, Password Plus by Milton Bradley. The patient needs to be able to read individual words. The object of the game is to give clues so that players can guess each other's word. The game can be made easier for the patient by allowing him to use clues of more than one word. 2–4 players.

Solitaire and Other Card Games

Solitaire card games. These card games are, by definition, those which can be played by one person. The patient must be able to recognize numbers and suits and must know their order from lowest to highest. There are many different types of these games. If the patient knew Solitaire games before his illness and enjoyed them, you might suggest his trying them again. If he has never played but is willing to try, find a book about Solitaire and choose games which are easy to learn.

Boxed card games. There are many of these available, and they usually have special cards and rules. Some are very easy to learn; others are more difficult. Some are basic matching games, but others may require number or spelling skills. Read the instructions on the package to see if you think that the patient is able to play it. Some examples are Flinch, Grabitz, Mille Bornes, Old Maid, Pit, Rummy, Uno, and Water Works.

Poker Keeno by Cadaco. If the patient is having difficulty recognizing cards or telling the suits apart, this is a good game to play. It is played with what looks like a Bingo card with small playing cards instead of numbers on it. The object is to cover five in a row like a Bingo card. Playing cards are announced (like numbers in Bingo) or the patient can match the cards by himself. 1 or more players.

Card games. If the patient enjoyed playing certain card games such as bridge, hearts, euchre, poker, and tripoly before his illness, he may want to try them again. Make sure that you begin slowly and allow him time to recall how each game is played. If he seems confused or frustrated, it might be better to simplify the game in some fashion or try another time.

Other Games

Things To Do Alone

The games and ideas which follow can be done alone. The patient may need help to start but should be able to continue independently. These are meant to be fun, and perhaps some of the ideas will appeal to him. You will need to determine which games might be too easy, too difficult, or boring. Your clinician can help with the choices.

Games that can be played alone. These games are taken from the ones mentioned earlier. They are listed here alphabetically because the patient can use them by himself. In some cases, you may need to change the rules slightly to permit one person to play alone.

Ad Lib, Perquackey, Scrabble Crossword Cubes Game, Spill and Spell (see page 159)
Bingo (see page 157)
Boggle, Big Boggle (see page 159)
Concentration (see page 157)
Dominoes (see page 156)
Facts in Five (see page 160)
Lotto (see page 156)
Memory Card Matching Game (see page 157)
Perfection, Superfection (see page 157)
Picture Tri-Ominos (see page 156)
Poker Keeno (see page 160)
Quad-Ominos (see page 156)
Scrabble Crossword Dominoes (see page 159)
Scrabble Sentence Cubes (see page 160)
Stack-Ominos (see page 156)
Trac 4 (see page 157)
Tri-Ominos (see page 156)
Yahtzee (see page 158)

Electronic learning games. The variety of electronic learning games or machines available to the public is increasing all the time. There are several that can be called "learning tools" and can be excellent for the aphasic person. Your clinician will help you decide which ones can be of value to your family member.

Electronic Learning Machine by Coleco. This has a changeable keyboard and many different activities, ranging from easy to fairly difficult.

Quiz Whiz by Coleco. You read questions from a book and answer them on the machine. The patient must be able to read well to use this.

Simon by Milton Bradley. This game works on memory skills by showing a pattern in four colors that the player tries to duplicate.

Speak and Math by Texas Instruments. This game has a number keyboard for practicing arithmetic skills.

Speak and Read by Texas Instruments. This game has an alphabet keyboard and several reading activities ranging from easy to difficult.

Speak and Spell by Texas Instruments. This game has an alphabet keyboard for working on spelling skills.

Spelling B by Texas Instruments. This game has a very small alphabet keyboard for practice in spelling common objects.

Electronic entertainment games. There are many varieties in the stores, some simple and inexpensive, some complex and very expensive. They range from small hand-held devices to video cartridges. In most of these, one person competes against a computer. There are also other varieties in which two people can play against each other. The patient may enjoy some of these, but he can become very frustrated if they prove too hard.

Crossword puzzle books or magazines. These games come in many levels of difficulty. There are some "easy" crossword magazines that you can try. Probably the best ones are children's crosswords, which may be appropriate for your family member. They can be found on magazine racks and among children's books. Your clinician can help you find the best ones for the patient.

Other word puzzles. There are magazines which offer pencil or word games, mazes, puzzle books, etc. Many of these are similar to crosswords, but others are very different (such as quizzes, anagrams, cryptograms, etc.). Book stores or drugstores often have puzzle or game sections. Ask your clinician if you are not sure what to buy.

Word Search, Word Find, Word Hunt, Search-a-Word. These puzzles are called many things and are listed separately because they are now popular. They are good for the patient who has spelling difficulties.

Yes and Know Invisible Ink Quiz and Game Books by Lee Publications. These particular books have a unique pen that uncovers "invisible" answers. The patient can play different games and quizzes by himself but may need help in understanding how to play the first time.

Quiz or brain-teaser books. There are books of this sort for both children and adults. They often have questions about subjects such as sports, TV, trivia, brain teasers, and riddles. These can range from relatively easy to very difficult. Check through a few pages to see if you think your family member will be able to handle the book or ask your clinician for advice.

Children's activity books. Children's books, especially those that are "learning" books, might also be interesting and challenging to the patient. Books stores and toy stores will sell these.

Small packaged puzzles for one person. These are too many to list individually. They are manufactured by many companies, and what is available will differ from one place to another. Some are three-dimensional, involving pieces which fit together into a shape of some sort. Some require a steady hand to move pieces in a certain way; some resemble miniature sports games or pinball machines; some use letters, numbers, pegs, balls, or water. Most stores with even a small toy section carry these types of puzzles.

Jigsaw puzzles. These come in many sizes and shapes. There are children's puzzles with very few pieces and others with up to two thousand pieces. Check the size and number of pieces before you make a purchase. If the puzzle is too hard, the patient may become very frustrated and give up.

TV game shows. The patient as a home viewer can try to guess the answers along with television contestants. The home versions of these games may be interesting for the patient if he watches the TV version and already knows how to play the game.

Drawing and painting kits, coloring and dot-to-dot books. The patient might enjoy trying one of these for fun and for coordination. Drawing or painting kits usually are found in craft departments or stores. Coloring or dot-to-dot books are usually found in stores in children's book or toy departments.

Hobby kits, craft kits. There are many types to choose from, and usually department or toy stores will have hobby or craft sections. Some examples of hobbies are collecting stamps or coins, electric trains, woodworking, refinishing furniture, collecting or making miniatures, flower arranging, and model cars. Some popular crafts are rug hooking, weaving, ceramics, making floral centerpieces, making candles, string art, macramé, and quilting.

Handwork. Both men and women can enjoy this sort of activity. Some examples are sewing, knitting, crocheting, crewel work, needlepoint, and embroidery. There are kits on the market, as well as classes, which can help someone learn the simplest or most complex skills. There are also devices to help a patient with only one usable hand.

Sports. There are non-strenuous sports which the aphasic person can perform by himself. Some examples are darts, bowling, miniature golf, billiards (pool), croquet, and horseshoes.

Other Things To Do Alone

COMMUNITY RESOURCES

Introduction

You might be surprised to learn that your community is ready to help in many ways. Various organizations and services may already exist to ease your burden. This section briefly discusses the community resources which you may find available.

Community organizations can help in two ways. They provide valuable assistance in solving problems affecting the aphasic person. Highly trained professionals as well as dedicated volunteers can offer a number of community-oriented services. In addition, they permit the patient to get out of the home into the community so that he can feel active and a part of society again. While some patients will not be able physically to function as they did in the past, any activities in which they do participate will help ease feelings of isolation and helplessness.

Of particular help are the aphasia social clubs and leisure and recreational programs. Aphasic persons will find that they are not alone in their limitations. They can learn that despite their aphasia, a rich experience is still possible.

Family members are urged to take full advantage of this section of the book and to seek out as many appropriate resources as possible.

M. R.

How To Use the Community Resources

This section is divided into ten possible areas of concern to the patient and family. Not all of the areas may be appropriate for everyone, but there may be several which you will want to explore.

Each area of concern is briefly described, and several suggestions are then given as to where to go or who to call for help.

These listings cannot be complete or totally accurate for the entire country. The sources most helpful in one place may not be useful in another. Some departments, organizations, or offices will have different names in different states. In some communities they may not exist, while in others the source may have several branches. For these reasons, alternative sources are discussed. In addition to the sources listed, your physician and speech-language pathologist should be able to help with some of your questions. Your local library and municipal offices may be helpful in answering questions about local programs.

In general, the sources are arranged so that those most likely to be of assistance are listed first. The right side of the page is left blank so that you can jot down phone numbers or make other notes. Your clinician may also add notes or suggestions for services with which he is familiar.

The last two areas of this section are slightly different from the others. Areas Related to Aphasia suggests some sources of help for situations which are often associated with aphasia. Aids for the Aphasic Patient suggests some items you may wish to consider to make life easier for the patient.

Funding for Rehabilitation Services

Rehabilitation services usually included as part of a team approach can include those of speech-language pathologists, physical therapists, occupational therapists, recreational therapists, and social workers. Most insurance policies cover these services if the patient is hospitalized, but there are usually limits or variations to the coverage when he is in another environment. This section suggests some sources for financial help for these kinds of rehabilitation services.

The first and most important thing to do is to check your insurance policy. Some Blue Cross/Blue Shield policies, major (or master) medical policies, and other insurance companies may pay for outpatient services that you or your family member might need.

If the policy is through your employer, check any papers you have for explanations of the policy, and talk to a supervisor or someone in your personnel department. You can also call a local or regional office of your insurance company and speak to someone about your policy and the type of service in which you are interested. If you do have coverage for the service, ask whether there are time or monetary limits to it and whether you can get this information in writing.

If you find that your particular policy will not provide money for the services you need or that you will be exceeding the limit of your coverage, you may find the following listings helpful.

Medicare. If the patient is over sixty-five or has been disabled for a certain period of time, he is eligible for Medicare benefits. Several rehabilitative services may be included, but the patient must be receiving treatment through a program that has been approved by Medicare for this service to be paid. You can learn more about Medicare benefits through your local Social Security office.

Medicaid. In many states this program will pay for rehabilitative services. If you do not have medical insurance, you may be eligible for Medicaid. This is not an automatic benefit, however, and your individual situation must be approved and reviewed periodically. Contact your county Department of Social Services to apply.

Department or Bureau of Vocational Rehabilitation, State Department of Education. This is a government-supported service. Its purpose is to help an individual return to some type of work environment. As a result, rehabilitation services may be partially or fully funded. You may be referred to this department or you may call yourself to set up an appointment with a counselor. There will be a central vocational rehabilitation office in your state capital. A listing of this resource is in your telephone book under your state listings.

Veterans Administration Services. Any veteran is eligible for benefits through a VA hospital. Aphasia rehabilitation and other services are usually offered at these facilities. If what the patient needs is not available, the Veterans Administration may pay for these services elsewhere.

Department of Social Work or Family Services in your county or hospital. If you need services which your insurance will not cover and which you cannot afford, you may be eligible for assistance through this

NOTES

department. Such departments have access to many resources and may be able to find the help or funding that you need. There is a social work or family services department in most hospitals; if not, there will be a county or local office which you can call.

Local service clubs. There are probably service groups active near you. These may be local chapters of national or regional clubs or local community service groups specific to your area. Each will have its own service projects which can differ within any chapter or club. Many are committed to helping the handicapped, which in some cases includes speech- and language-impaired (and aphasic) adults. Examples of clubs interested in the communicatively impaired include the Jaycees, Kiwanis, Lions, Optimists, and Sertoma. Some may be involved with certain service programs and some may consider individual cases. Talk with your physician, speech-language pathologist, social worker, or someone involved in the organization for more information.

National organizations. Some nationwide organizations use a portion of their funds for rehabilitation services. Examples of these are the Easter Seal Society, the Sister Kenny Institute, and the United Fund. Easter Seal operates some of its own rehabilitation service programs, and fees are variable. Sister Kenny and United Fund may support rehabilitation services within hospital or clinical programs. Ask any of your health care professionals or call the organization for information on activities in your area.

NOTES

Other Sources of Information

Home-Bound Care

Some aphasic persons may not be able to leave the house, and so may require medical and/or rehabilitative services at home. The patient in a wheelchair or confined to bed may need home care services. The patient who is unable to get to rehabilitation services because of transportation problems may also qualify for home care.

The following list provides some sources that can help you to find people to come to your home. Your insurance may pay for some or all of this type of care. You may also need an order from your physician to receive some services. If you are not directly referred, you can locate the sources in your telephone book.

Visiting Nurse Association. This nation-wide group employs a variety of home health care personnel including nurses, therapists, and speech-language pathologists.

Home health care services or agencies. Many states sponsor both community and private health care agencies which employ health care professionals.

NOTES

Private practitioners. These include
nurses, nurses' aides, physical or occupational therapists, and speech-language pathologists. They may be self-employed or
may work for an agency, and not all of
them may be willing to come to your
home. Ask for referrals from other professionals or look in the classified ads of
your local newspaper.
Your county Public Health Department.
This department may provide services or
may refer you to those who can.
Your hospital. Some hospitals may provide home care services or may have
someone on the staff who will help you
locate what you need. If your family
member has been in the hospital, check
with your physician or the hospital staff
to find these services.

Other Sources of Information

Transportation Services

Sometimes it is difficult to arrange transportation for appointments, errands, shopping, or just visiting. Some sources for finding transportation if you do not have a driver and do not drive yourself are suggested below. Your first step is to ask friends and relatives to help you.

Volunteer drivers. There may be people who are willing to help by providing rides on a temporary or permanent basis. Perhaps you know of or can find someone who can provide transportation at least one way. Perhaps there is someone living near you who regularly goes to the same hospital or clinic that you do and with whom you can share a ride. Some hospital or rehabilitation service programs offer volunteer drivers.

Volunteer services in your community. A volunteer service organization or bureau may exist which provides transportation for those who are homebound. Your local or county offices or senior citizen groups can help you locate these services.

Local transportation systems. Some communities have small buses or vans that transport people within certain boundaries. Such a system may be called a Dial-a-Ride system. Check with your municipal offices to see if these are available to you. Bus or taxi service may also be available.

Ethnic or religious organizations. Your place of worship may supply volunteer drivers. If you are a member of a minority group, there may be agencies to help you. Call your county government offices for information.

Associations that service a particular illness. If you or your family member has an illness in addition to aphasia, contact an appropriate organization such as the Heart Association or the Cancer Society. These are listed in the telephone book and they may have drivers to help you.

NOTES

**Transportation services for the handi-
capped.** A person with aphasia or someone who cannot drive because of a health
problem is usually eligible for this kind of
service. Check with your local or county
transportation offices to see what is available in your area.

Hire a driver. The classified ads or Yellow Pages may have a list of licensed, in-
sured people who will drive for a fee.
Another alternative is to offer to pay
friends, neighbors, or relatives for a ride.
See **Volunteer Help** opposite. You can
use these sources for help with transportation problems.

NOTES

Other Sources of Information

Volunteer Help

You may find that you are unable to leave the aphasic person alone at home. If this is a problem, you may need extra help: someone who is medically trained for health care, someone trained in rehabilitation work, someone to run errands, someone to help with household chores, or someone just to be with the patient while you are out.

The following list gives some ideas of how to locate volunteer help. If a medically or professionally trained person is needed, the section on Home-Bound Care will probably be more valuable than this one.

Relatives, friends, and neighbors. They may be willing to help but unsure about what they can do. They may appreciate specific suggestions on how they can help.

Volunteer groups. People who volunteer their services on a regular basis may be available in your community. They may be willing to donate some time in a number of ways. Retired professionals or volunteers with special skills are sometimes willing to go to homes to help with care, exercises, housework, driving, etc. If you have a community services directory, look in this. Your local library or municipal offices may also have information.

Ethnic or religious organizations. These groups often have volunteers to help those in need. If you are a member of a minority group or a religious organization, call its main office for assistance.

Hospital or medical center. You can contact the place where your family member was a patient, where your doctor is on the staff, or where you would ordinarily go for out-patient treatment. Some hospitals or medical centers have volunteer services that may be able to help you.

Associations that serve a particular illness. If you qualify, this kind of organization may be able to help. Examples include your state Heart Association and Cancer Society. They are listed in the telephone book.

NOTES

Local service clubs. Some examples are the Elks, Jaycees, Junior League, Kiwanis, Lions, and Masons. In addition to providing help to their own members, these organizations serve individuals with special needs, such as senior citizens, the blind, and the speech-impaired and hearing-impaired. You will need to check with your health care professional or the chapters in your area for more information.

Adult community education programs and senior citizen groups. Someone associated with adult education programs may be aware of volunteers. Homebound teachers or individuals with specialized skills willing to share their time may be available. Community senior citizen groups may also have persons interested in helping others. Your library, education, or municipal offices may know who to contact.

High school or college students, and neighbors. They may be interested in volunteering to help you. Students may be able to get credit for a class or project, may want experience, or may have a personal interest in aphasia.

Boy Scouts, Girl Scouts, and Campfire Girls. Individual troops may have volunteer projects. Some individuals may need to volunteer their services to receive a "bar" or award. Call a local or county office to inquire about a troop near you.

Other sources. Municipal offices, a community service directory, "help" lines (the names vary and can be run by radio, telephone, or television organizations), community, school, or store bulletin boards, and neighborhood newsletters are example of other sources which can help.

NOTES

Other Sources of Information

Counseling Services

When a loved one suddenly experiences aphasia and its related difficulties, the impact on the family unit can be devastating. Life is disrupted in a way that you have probably never experienced before. Adjusting to and understanding these changes are important aspects of rehabilitation for the patient and his family. Feelings such as depression, guilt, fear, anger, frustration, denial, and helplessness are common for both patient and family members. Talking over these feelings and hearing or reading about others who have been through the same thing is often comforting; however, many families find that additional professional help is beneficial.

Psychiatrists, psychologists, psychotherapists, and social workers are all professionals trained to support and help you and your family through this difficult time. Your family physician or any other health care professional with whom you are working can suggest the type of counselor best suited to your needs. You can also ask them to recommend specific individuals or programs.

If you do not have a recommendation or referral, the groups listed below usually offer counseling services to individuals. The Yellow Pages has listings which may be helpful.

**Department of Social Work or Family
Services in your hospital or medical facility.** Some departments provide counseling as one of their services. Even if a
department does not, it will be able to refer you to other sources.

**Community or family service organiza-
tions.** The names vary from place to
place, but the concept is the same: to
provide help. This usually includes counseling services. Your municipal offices or
community services directory can help
you locate a family service organization in
your area.

Religious family service organizations.
Catholic Social Service, Jewish Family
Service, and similar organizations usually
have trained counselors (often social
workers). If you are interested, they may
be of help.

NOTES

Other Sources of Information

Retesting of Driving Skills

You may wonder whether or not the aphasic person can or should drive again. In some cases it is simply a matter of when the person feels ready to drive, but in many cases a number of other factors, including state laws, are involved.

A general rule is to ask your doctor first. Other persons whose opinions will be valuable in determining driving readiness will be physical and occupational therapists and your ophthalmologist, neurologist, physiatrist, and speech-language pathologist. Questions about physical limitations, visual field and/or visual perceptual abilities, reflexes, judgment, and reaction times are all important considerations.

The four sources listed below have professionals to help evaluate the patient's driving skills.

Rehabilitation institutes or centers. These usually have staff members who are certified to evaluate people for driving. They will be familiar with problems of aphasia and/or paralysis.

Department of Vocational Rehabilitation, State Department of Education. This agency employs vocational counselors who know how to help you with information and decisions about driving. Look under your state listings in the telephone book.

Department of Transportation, Secretary of State's office, or wherever you go to renew your driver's license. This office may have someone qualified to test your family member. The office can also help the patient pass the necessary tests even if he cannot read or write.

Private driving instructors. Many are qualified to make a judgment on driving abilities in addition to giving driving lessons. They are listed in the Yellow Pages.

NOTES

Other Sources of Information

Vocational Planning

Some people will never be able to return to work because of aphasia and/or related medical problems. Other people will be able to return to some kind of employment—but not to their original jobs. Some will be able to return to their jobs but may require some changes in responsibility. In general, those who find a change in occupation necessary may find vocational counseling helpful. Some places to contact for professional guidance are listed below.

Department of Vocational Rehabilitation, State Department of Education. These counselors are trained to help you make decisions regarding your job, employment opportunities, and work benefits, and provide other services as well. The bureau is listed in the telephone book under your state listing.

NOTES

Vocational counselors employed in a rehabilitation center. They may be part of a team and qualified to help you with employment questions. You usually do not need to be a patient in such a center in order to have an interview.

Community vocational advisors or counselors. They may be working privately, or for insurance companies; they are listed in the Yellow Pages. They can provide vocational testing and counseling.

NOTES

Other Sources of Information

Stroke and Aphasia Clubs

Stroke and aphasia clubs are active in many places around the country. These clubs range from support groups headed by professionals to informal social groups that meet for monthly dinners. Some groups are recreational and meet several days a week. Others are located in a speech and language center or in someone's home. These groups are growing in number nationwide because of the important part they play in the lives of the aphasic person and his family.

The following list gives some suggestions for finding a club in your area.

Your state Heart Association. This organization sponsors stroke and aphasia clubs around the nation. Call your state or local branch for information.

Department of Social Services of your county, hospital, rehabilitation, or community health service. This department may be able to give you information on local clubs or direct you to a source of help.

Speech and language pathology services in a clinic, university, hospital, nursing home, office, or rehabilitation center. They will be aware of clubs in the area or may have groups or their own.

Your city or county Department of Parks and Recreation. Some communities have stroke and aphasia recreation groups that are run through this local department.

Senior citizen groups. At times, stroke and aphasia groups combine programs with senior citizen groups. Check with local groups to see if this is true in your area.

Other Sources of Information

NOTES

Leisure and Recreational Activities

The aphasic patient faces a change in his lifestyle. It may be temporary or permanent. Readjustments and changes may be major or only minor. These changes affect not just the patient but all members of the family as well.

Very often a patient will become bored and irritable because of the forced change in routine. He may need alternative ways to spend his time. The suggestions which follow provide some ideas.

Stroke clubs: There may be several sponsors of these clubs—the American Heart Association, speech and language clinics, hospitals, universities, communities, and professional people. They can be most valuable in helping the patient meet other people who are facing similar situations. Although not all groups are alike, their aims are mainly social, educational, or recreational. Your speech-language pathologist may be aware of a club near you (see pp. 179–80).

Senior citizen groups. More and more communities are starting these groups, which can include meetings, crafts, games, exercise, meals, and trips. They can be very informal get-togethers and may vary as to age requirements. Sometimes stroke and aphasia patients are welcome, sometimes not. Some groups are only for men, others only for women, others mixed. Your city hall, city recreation director, adult education director, or library can help you find a group in your area.

Recreational programs. Usually these are offered through adult education services. Sometimes schools provide a gym or pool for adults. Sometimes there are classes for those with medical problems or physical limitations. Call your city hall, Department of Parks and Recreation, or adult education director for information.

Recreational therapy. This is usually available through your hospital or rehabilitation center (see p. 189).

NOTES

Parks or nature programs. If you have a local or regional park, recreation, or nature center, it may have programs such as walks, bird watching, lectures, etc. You can contact the park, your city office, or the regional Department of Parks and Recreation.

Health clubs. There are several chains of health clubs as well as private organizations which will have gyms, exercise rooms, pools, jogging tracks, tennis, and racquetball. They will usually provide individualized programs. Check with the patient's doctor before he starts something of this type.

Veterans Administration. If your family member qualifies as a veteran, he may be entitled to benefits. In addition to speech and language pathology services, many VA hospitals sponsor social, recreational, or family support groups.

Art and craft classes. Many aphasic patients have learned to enjoy a new hobby and have also learned to do it one-handed if necessary. You can find out about different classes available through community adult education programs, local schools, senior citizen groups, craft stores, private advertising (bulletin boards, newspapers, flyers), or word of mouth. Sometimes there are special classes for the handicapped which aphasics may attend. There are also many craft or hobby kits on the market which the patient might like.

Community adult education programs. These classes are becoming more popular all over the country. Some may be appropriate for family members, others for the patient himself. Check with your clinician or an instructor if you are not sure whether your family member should enroll.

Classes for the handicapped. The speech- or language-impaired person may be eligible to register for these classes. These

NOTES

may help the patient learn a new skill, take short outings, work through individual problems, exercise, and socialize. Contact the community adult education programs, vocational rehabilitation services, or a physical, occupational, or recreational therapist.

Libraries. Many libraries have collections of books and magazines in large print. They may also have tape or record collections which may be of interest to the patient.

National Library Service for the Blind and Physically Handicapped. If the patient is not able to read but understands all that is said to him, he may be eligible for this service. The headquarters are in Washington, D.C., but there are many participating libraries around the country. It is a "talking library" of current magazines and books on cassette, tapes, or special records. They can be borrowed or sent to your home on a regular basis. Your local librarian can tell you how to apply.

Hobbies. This may be a good time to revive an old hobby or begin a new one. Gardening, playing an instrument, joining a club, taking care of a pet, or collecting something may be appealing and enjoyable for the patient (p. 164).

Volunteer work. The patient may be capable of work despite some limitations. All communities appreciate volunteer help in schools, hospitals, homes, churches, and other organizations. If you are unsure what the patient can do, check with your therapists to see whether they have some suggestions.

Ethnic or religious organizations. There may be activities or groups suited for the family or the patient. Check with the appropriate source about what is available.

YMCA, YWCA. These organizations may have programs for the aphasic patient.

NOTES

Games and other pastimes. Section II of
this book has ideas for things to do. Perhaps the patient will be interested in trying some of them.

Music therapy. Music therapists can work
independently or for a health care facility. They use music in a variety of ways
and can explore what would be appropriate for each patient. These therapists can
develop programs to fit the needs and
skills of each patient.

Other Sources of Information

Home Aids for the Patient

The examples of aids which follow may be helpful to you and the
patient. These are items which can be bought or made to help make
his life easier. They have been used by other aphasic persons and
found to be helpful. They are not going to be appropriate for all
patients, but you may find ideas for your family member.

Aids for the physically impaired. Physical difficulties will vary with
each patient—from a slight facial weakness to paralysis of one side of
the body. There are aids available for almost any type of difficulty.
When you identify the problem, your physician may have some suggestions, and the books listed on page 198 may offer other ideas. If
your doctor has ordered physical and/or occupational therapy, the
therapists will also be able to give you help. They will have catalogs
with devices you can order.

Bedside tables. The typical hospital bedside table has legs on one side that extend under the bed. These can be purchased for your home. There are some which tilt in several directions and some which adjust in height. Any table used should be at a convenient height and be fairly stable.

Bed trays. If the patient is confined to bed or a couch, these trays may be helpful. They have short legs which rest on the mattress while the tray fits over the person's legs, providing a table on which to eat, read, write, place things, etc.

Bell. If the patient is confined to a room, it may be difficult for him to call those in other rooms. If a bell is available he can ring it to get attention.

Book or page holders. These items hold books upright and open to a certain page. (Some are intended for cookbooks, for example.) These will let the patient read a page without having to hold the book himself. You can also buy holders for playing cards if the patient has difficulty holding them.

Chalkboard. A chalkboard set up somewhere in the home can make a good message center. It can easily be erased and the messages changed. It may be easier for a patient to write on a chalkboard than on paper if he is having trouble forming letters. Messages can be written in large print if he has trouble reading. When things to do are listed on the board, he can erase each one as it is completed.

Clipboard. The patient should have something hard on which to write. A clipboard is easy to carry around and may have attached containers in which to store supplies.

Clock with movable hands. This can be a large children's toy clock with hands that move. It may be helpful to remind the patient of the time when he needs to do something, such as taking a pill, making a phone call or putting something in the oven. The toy clock can be set for the patient to compare with a working clock.

Daily schedule. It may be helpful to write the date at the top of a sheet of paper and then list the things that the patient will be doing on a particular day (he can make the list if he is able to write). It can include things such as appointments, chores, medications, and instructions.

Driving conveniences. These may be helpful if the patient has some paralysis, has difficulty getting in and out of the car, or needs special devices for driving. A physical or occupational therapist can help you find the right equipment. Vocational rehabilitation counselors as well as the counselors found wherever you go to renew your driver's license can also be of assistance.

Emergency alarms. These can be installed anywhere in a home for emergency situations. One type of emergency alarm is a button which is put next to a bed, in the kitchen, etc. It can be wired directly to an ambulance, police or fire station, or neighbor's or relative's house. If the button is pushed, a telephone will ring and a tape-recorded message will play. Another type is worn by the patient himself. It too is wired so that if the patient pushes the device a message is transmitted to the sources of help.

Emergency list. It may be a good idea to make a list of important phone numbers (police, fire, neighbor, relative, etc.) and leave them near the telephone. If the numbers are needed in a hurry, the patient does not have to remember them or look them up in a telephone book.

Exercising devices. You should check with the patient's doctor before you look into anything of this kind. There are many exercising devices available, such as the stationary bicycle.

Fact sheet. If the patient is fairly independent but has trouble remembering or communicating, he might find it helpful to have a fact sheet to carry and refer to. It can include important telephone numbers, vital statistics, social security number, bank and account numbers, driver's license number, and any other personal information. If he does much check-writing but sometimes has trouble with numbers, a small card with the numbers spelled out may be helpful.

Hearing amplifiers. These are different from hearing aids. Most are either held in the hand or used with earphones. They are used for a short period of time; they make noises and voices louder to the person using them.

Household aids. If the patient has a weakness or paralysis of some kind, these may be helpful. There are many aids and devices available. (See page 184.)

Identification card. If the patient has trouble communicating, he might benefit by carrying a card that you can make. It can list his name, address, telephone number, an explanation that he has a speech problem, and any other useful information.

Lap desk. This is a writing surface for someone who is not sitting at a table. On one side it has a hard surface attached to a pillow. The soft pillow underneath does not cramp the legs, and the hard surface is easy to write on.

Large calendar. If the patient has a number of appointments or events each week, a large calendar may be filled out ahead of time and displayed somewhere at home.

Large print materials. There are books and magazines published in large print (see page 183). If the larger print is helpful to the patient, then you might also use large letters and a bold felt-tip pen when you write.

Magnetic board. Large letters and numbers can be bought to use for messages with this board. If the patient is having spelling problems, it may help him to have letters to look at when he puts together a word or message. The letters are large enough for someone who has trouble grasping to use.

Magnifying glass. If the patient seems to be having difficulty with small print or has some other visual problem, a magnifying glass might help. The familiar round ones come in several sizes and strengths. Some look like rulers and enlarge a line of print. Others have lights on them, and others fit over regular glasses. The patient should try several to see what is best for him.

Messages. A central place for family messages will let the patient know where to look for a message and where to leave one. If paper and pencil are stored there, he will know where to find them.

Paper. It may be helpful to have paper and pencil handy for the patient to reach if he wants to try writing, drawing, practicing, or doodling. Lined paper may be helpful if he is having trouble forming the letters or writing on a straight line.

Pill boxes. If the patient has to take pills on a set schedule, there are pill boxes designed to help in several ways. Some have compartments for different pills, some are set up like a clock with compartments that correspond to the hours of the day, and some have alarms which ring when it is time to take a pill.

Pillow. If the patient will be sitting up in bed or on a couch, his back will need support. Some pillows are self-supporting, so that he can lean against them while sitting. Some have "arms" on which he can lean, and some have built-in pockets.

Protection devices. There are several types of protection devices on the market. Two common ones are carried in a pocket or purse: one contains a chemical to squirt into an attacker's face, and the other sends out a very loud "scream."

Special watches. If the patient is having trouble telling time, there are special digital watches available. Some patients may find hands easier to read, while others may prefer the digital numbers. Some watches have built-in alarms that can be pre-set to go off at certain times.

Tape-recorded material. There are books and magazines recorded on cassette tape (see page 183). If this is helpful to the patient, you can use tape-recorded messages for other purposes too.

Tape recorder. This is helpful in order to remember conversations. At work or class there may be important facts to remember which the patient may not be able to write down. For example he might record and then replay his doctor's comments and instructions.

Telephone devices. Several types of devices are available to make it easier for persons with communication problems to use the telephone. If the patient has difficulty remembering or writing down phone messages, a telephone-answering device lets him listen to a message as many times as he wants. Another device lets you "program" specific telephone numbers into your phone system. Any name you want programmed is written next to one button, which the patient pushes in order to make the call. Telephone companies and some stores sell these, and your speech-language pathologist or physical or occupational therapist may have some additional suggestions.

Writing utensils. If the patient is having difficulty with his handwriting because of a muscular weakness, he may find some writing utensils easier to use than others. Sometimes certain penpoints or felt-tip markers are easier to use than others. A soft lead pencil (No. 2) may be easier to use than a hard one, and a fat writing utensil may be easier to grasp and control than a regular-sized one. If he is using a pencil, have erasers available for him.

Other Suggestions

Areas Related to Aphasia

The first four listings in this section represent services which, along with speech-language pathology, are usually considered part of a team approach to rehabilitation. Some patients may benefit from all of these, some will not. They are available at most hospitals and medical or rehabilitation centers and at some nursing homes and extended care facilities. These professionals, along with your physician, will be happy to help you with your questions and problems—feel free to ask them.

There are some conditions which are often associated with aphasia. They are separate from the speech or language impairment but often occur along with it. This section goes on to mention them. It is suggested that you look over all this material to find whatever information is most useful to you.

Physical therapy. Physical therapists use treatments and exercises for strengthening and coordinating muscles which are not working properly. You will need a referral from your doctor to begin this kind of therapy. You can also see a physiatrist (a medical doctor specializing in rehabilitation medicine) who will determine whether physical therapy can benefit your family member.

Occupational therapy. Like physical therapists, occupational therapists work on strengthening and coordinating muscle movements. They are especially helpful in showing patients the best way to handle everyday tasks such as dressing, bathing, and cooking. You will need a referral from your doctor or a physiatrist for this therapy.

Recreational therapy. Recreational therapists help individuals develop recreational interests and encourage them to participate in different types of activities. They are usually a part of rehabilitation services.

Social work. Social workers may help the family or patient in such ways as working for a smooth transition from a medical to home environment, emotional support and counseling, and general problem-solving. If there is a social services department in your medical facility, you can usually use its services even after the patient is at home.

Exercise. A regular exercise program is usually an important part of rehabilitation, especially if physical impairments are present. Your doctor will know how much exercise and what type is advisable for your family member. Be sure to check with him before the patient starts any daily exercise periods, health club programs, or recreational activities. If the patient is getting physical therapy, he may be asked to practice some specific exercises that have been prescribed for him.

Nutrition and diet. Your doctor is the best person to contact if you have questions about this. He may suggest that you see a dietician or nutritionist to help you plan meals, particularly if the patient should be on a special diet.

Medications and vitamins. Your doctor can determine whether the patient should be taking vitamins. If you have questions about any medications, ask your doctor or pharmacist. It is important for your doctors to know all medications that the patient has been taking, and also that he is taking them exactly as directed.

Swallowing or digestive problems. Your doctor, nurse, and speech-language pathologist will be aware of these problems. If there are any sudden changes, contact one of them immediately.

Bowel and bladder functioning. If you have any questions about this, contact your doctor. He should be aware of any changes that may occur in these habits. If there are nurses helping to care for the patient, tell one of them about your concerns.

Emotional or coping difficulties. These are commonly associated with family members as well as with the patient. See the section on counseling services, pp. 175–76.

Sexual difficulties. It is common to experience changes in sexual functioning which can be emotional, medical, or physical in nature, and which may involve either partner. Talking to your doctor and to other health care and rehabilitation specialists may be helpful. Counselors (especially those involved with rehabilitation) are knowledgeable about normal sexual changes after stroke or aphasia and will discuss these matters with you.

Visual problems. The patient may think that his vision is worse than it was before his aphasia. This may only appear to be the case and may not indicate a need for glasses or a change in prescription. These difficulties usually improve as time goes on. Ophthalmologists are medically trained and able to recognize whether the problems are related to the brain injury or to an actual loss of vision. Your doctor may recommend that you wait a period of time before you see an ophthalmologist in order to allow the major changes of the eyes to take place.

Hearing problems. The patient may think that his hearing is worse than it was before his aphasia. This may be related to the aphasic difficulties rather than to an actual hearing loss. Often speech and language pathology services are provided in the same location with audiologists (hearing specialists), so this can be checked very easily.

Other Suggestions

SUGGESTED READING LIST

Introduction

In most instances, the more we know about a problem, the better we can deal with it. Finding good reading material about aphasia, however, has not always been easy. This section contains a list of readings to help you understand the problems of aphasia.

Many of the publications on the list have been written by aphasic patients who have recovered. These will be especially helpful in understanding how aphasia is affecting your family member. The fears and frustrations of having lost the ability to speak, read, or write need special attention. Understanding and patience are vitally important.

The author has taken special care to select publications useful in explaining the effects of aphasia and its impact. Many of the items on the list discuss how aphasia affects personality, behavior, and emotions. Each selection is followed by a short description to help you decide whether it will be of interest.

It is known that certain aphasic patients may benefit from reading appropriate articles when they have recovered adequate reading skills. There is comfort in the knowledge that others are experiencing similar problems.

Family members are urged to learn all they can about aphasia from those who live with it, treat it, and describe its many forms.

M. R.

How To Use the Suggested Reading List

The books, articles, and pamphlets in this listing were chosen from more than ninety publications about aphasia. It was felt that these would be the most helpful to families who have not had previous experience with aphasia.

The readings provide information to help you understand and cope with aphasia. Some were written by professionals, others by people who have experienced aphasia at first hand or by spouses of those with aphasia. All selections are for the nonprofessional, and none are scientific in nature.

Most titles are followed by a paragraph that briefly explains their point of view. The author and publisher are included to help you find the publication. Additional readings are included if you want more readings or if some on the main list are not available.

If you wish to locate one of the books, there are several sources that you can use. Local libraries may carry some of the books. If they don't, they may be able to borrow some from another library. The journal articles can be found in some college or university libraries. The pamphlets can usually be ordered for a small fee from the organizations which publish them. Your speech-language pathologist may have some of these titles and other readings as well.

The last page of this section lists some books that might be of interest to those persons who have physical difficulties, more specifically, a right- or left-sided weakness. These books suggest how to manage a particular kind of physical handicap. They are not, however, as concerned with aphasia as are the other books.

Readings on Aphasia

About Stroke. Sister Kenny Institute, Rehabilitation Publication 724, Minneapolis, 1978. 38 pages.
> This pamplet answers questions about strokes. It explains some causes and possible effects and addresses some of the physical and emotional aspects of a stroke as well as the speech and language problems.

An Adult Has Aphasia. Daniel Boone, Interstate Publishers, Danville, Illinois, revised 1976. 24 pages.
> Written by a respected speech-language pathologist, the pamphlet offers an overview of aphasia. It is written for family members who want explanations of aphasia and suggestions for coping with it.

Aftermath of a Stroke. Robert Vincent Penney, Vantage Press, New York, 1978.
> Written by a 37-year-old physicist who had a stroke and aphasia and lost the use of his right arm, the book relates a story of his emotional and personal readjustments.

Aphasia, My World Alone. Helen Harlan Wulf, Wayne State University Press, Detroit, revised 1979.
> This woman experienced a stroke and aphasia. Her account is insightful, and provides an understanding of what an aphasic person is experiencing. She writes about some of the emotions, thoughts, and difficulties which she faced. This is the only item in this list written by a woman with aphasia.

Aphasia and the Family. American Heart Association, publication #50-002-A, Dallas, 1969. 24 pages.

This booklet provides information for the family about what aphasia is, how the family can help, and how to improve the patient's language.

"Aphasia as Seen by an Aphasic." Michael Rolnick and Ray Hoops, *Journal of Speech and Hearing Disorders*, volume 34, no. 1, 1969, pp. 48–53.

The speech-language pathologists who wrote this article interviewed six aphasic persons and explained their thoughts and experiences.

"An Aphasic's Reactions to His Communication Problems." Michael I. Rolnick and Carl Koski, *Journal of Communication Pathology*, volume 3, February 1969, pp. 1–6.

Carl Koski had an aneurysm that ruptured when he was 32, and the result was aphasia. He talks about his speech, reading, writing, and problems with understanding.

Comeback: The Story of My Stroke. Robert E. Van Rosen, Bobbs-Merrill Co., New York, 1963.

The author tells of his experiences with two strokes, aphasia, and a right-sided weakness. A section of the book gives some causes for a stroke, lists famous people who have had strokes (and aphasia), and offers some suggestions for how to do things one-handed.

Communication Problems after a Stroke. Sister Kenny Institute, Rehabilitation Publication 709, Minneapolis, 1978. 26 pages.

This pamphlet gives an overview of the problems that can occur following a stroke, including aphasia, paralysis, and emotional concerns.

Coping with Stroke (formerly *Communication Breakdown of Brain Injured Adults*). Helen Broida, College-Hill Press, Houston, 1979.

The author is a speech-language pathologist who works with aphasic adults. The book consists of questions which family members might ask a professional. The answers will help one understand aphasia and its related problems.

"Expressed Attitudes of Families of Aphasics." Russell L. Malone, *Journal of Speech and Hearing Disorders*, volume 34, May 1969, pp. 146–50.

Interviews were held with family members of twenty persons with aphasia. The article is concerned primarily with the feelings of these family members.

"An Open Letter to the Family of an Adult Patient with Aphasia." Betty Horowitz, *Rehabilitation Literature*, May 1962, pp. 141–44.

A speech-language pathologist has written an introduction for family members who are experiencing aphasia for the first time. The article consists of a list of do's and don't's and general suggestions.

"A Personal Account of Dysphasia." L. Sies and R. Butler, *Journal of Speech and Hearing Disorders*, volume 28, August 1963, pp. 261–66.

This article may be hard to find, but it gives a good account of a young man who was in a motorcycle accident. The descriptions of his feelings and some of his problems are interesting.

Portrait of Aphasia. David Knox, Wayne State University Press, Detroit, 1971. The husband of a woman who had aphasia from a stroke explains some of his wife's problems and how they both dealt with them. This is the only item in this list written by the husband of a woman with aphasia.

Silent Victory. Carmen McBride, Nelson-Hall Company, Chicago, 1969. The author wrote about her husband's aphasia during the two years before his death. He had a limited ability to communicate, and his wife tells their story. This is the only item in this list written by the wife of a man with aphasia.

Stroke: A Doctor's Personal Story of His Recovery. Charles Clay Dahlberg and Joseph Kaffe, W. W. Norton and Co., New York, 1977. Dr. Dahlberg was a psychiatrist and university professor who had a stroke with aphasia, but he returned to his practice and wrote about his experiences. Although he made an excellent recovery, he points out some of the difficulties that he went through. The book contains some technical information.

Stroke: A Guide for Patients and Their Families. John E. Sarno, M.D., and Martha Taylor Sarno, McGraw-Hill Book Co., New York, revised 1979. Martha Sarno is a respected aphasia clinician and John Sarno is a physician. Their book is written in question-and-answer format and includes all of the typical questions that someone wondering about stroke and aphasia might ask.

"Stroke: Some Psychological Problems It Causes." Frederick Whitehouse, M.D., *American Journal of Nursing,* October 1963, pp. 81–87. Although this article was written for nurses, it gives information about and descriptions of some of the social, personal, and behavioral changes which can occur with stroke and aphasia.

Stroke: A Study of Recovery. Douglas Ritchie, Doubleday and Co., New York, 1961. The author has written a diary account of his stroke and aphasia.

Stroke: Why Do They Behave That Way? American Heart Association, publication #50-035-A, Dallas. 32 pages. Two professors of psychology have written about some of the behaviors and common emotional stresses associated with stroke. They discuss them and give suggestions for coping with these difficulties.

A Stroke in the Family. Valerie Eaton Griffith, Delacorte Press, New York, 1970. This book was written by a friend of the actress Patricia Neal, who had aphasia after a stroke. It describes their day-to-day routine and activities.

Understanding Aphasia: A Guide for Medical and Paramedical Professionals. William Haynes and B. Greenberg, Interstate Publishers, New York, 1976. The typical problems facing an aphasic patient and his family are discussed. The subtitle indicates the audience to which the book is addressed. This is a more technical book than some of the others.

Other Suggested Readings

Additional Readings

This listing includes accounts of aphasia, as well as some general information.

"Aphasia According to an Expert." Mary Pannbacker, *Rehabilitation Literature,* volume 32, October 1971, pp. 295–98, 307.

Cry Babel. April Oursler Armstrong, Doubleday and Co., New York, 1979.

Dysphasia. McKenzie Buck, Prentice-Hall Inc., Englewood Cliffs, N.J., 1968.

Episode. Eric Hodgins, Atheneum, New York, 1964.

Heart Attack. Louis Levine, Harper and Row, New York, 1976.

"Patients Recovering from Aphasia Seek Understanding." Norma S. Stokes, *Modern Nursing Home,* September 1970, pp. 44–48.

Physiological and Psychological Considerations in the Management of Stroke. Arnold Brown, Warren H. Green, Inc., St. Louis, 1976.

Recovery with Aphasia. C. Scott Moss, University of Illinois Press, Urbana, 1972.

The Third Killer: Meditations on a Stroke. Guy Wint, Abelard-Schumann Ltd., New York, 1967.

Readings on Physical Handicaps

Aids to Independent Living. Edward Lowman and Judith Lannefield Klinger, McGraw-Hill Book Co., New York, 1969.

Care of the Patient with a Stroke. Genevieve Waples Smith, Springer Publishing Co., New York, 1976.

Do It Yourself Again. American Heart Association, publication #50-005-A, Dallas, 1969. 47 pages.

Hanging On. Hila Colman, Atheneum, New York, 1977.

Help Yourselves. Peggy E. Jay et al., Butterworth and Co., London, 1972.

How to Recover from a Stroke and Make a Successful Comeback. Clarence Longenecker, Ashley Books Inc., Port Washington, N.Y., 1977.

The One-Handers Book. Veronica Washam, John Day Co., New York, 1973.

Sourcebook for the Disabled. Edited by Glorya Hale, Paddington Press Ltd., London, 1979.

The organizations below publish pamphlets for those learning to live with physical handicaps. Ask your clinician or librarian about them or write for a list of their publications.

Institute of Rehabilitation Medicine
400 East 34th St.
New York, N.Y.   10016

Sister Kenny Institute
Abbott-Northwestern Hospital, Inc.
Publications-Audiovisuals Office #301
Chicago Ave. at 27th St.
Minneapolis, Minnesota   55407

SMALL OBJECTS

The following are examples of small objects you might find around the house for use in the activities.

Bathroom items: after-shave lotion, Band-Aids, bobby pin, brush, comb, cosmetics (lipstick, powder, rouge, mascara), dental floss, deodorant, electric shaver, false teeth, hair roller or curler, hair spray, hand lotion, medicines (pills, aspirin, cough syrup), mouthwash, nail file, nail clippers, perfume or cologne, razor blade, shampoo, shaving cream, soap, toothbrush, toothpaste, towel, washcloth

Clothing and jewelry: belt, bracelet, cuff link, earring, glove, handkerchief, hat, hosiery, necklace, necktie, pin, ring, scarf, shoe, shoelace, sock, tie bar, umbrella, watch

Desk items: address book, chalk, checkbook, crayon, envelope, felt-tip pen, file card, glue, letter opener, note pad, paper clip, paperweight, pen, pencil, rubber band, ruler, scissors, Scotch tape, stamp, stapler

Foods: cake mixes, candy, cereal, crackers, flour, fruit, jelly, ketchup, macaroni, mustard, nuts, olives, peanut butter, pepper, pet foods (dog biscuits, bird seed), pickles, popcorn, pudding, raisins, rice, salad dressing, salt, spaghetti, sugar, vegetables

Kitchen items: blender, bottle or can opener, bowl, cup, dish towel, drinking glass, fork, egg beater, knife, measuring cup, measuring spoon, mug, pans, plate, pitcher, pots, saucer, spatula, sponge, spoon, strainer, straw, tea kettle

Miscellaneous items: artificial flowers, ashtray, battery, bolt, calculator, camera, candle, Christmas ornaments, cigar, cigarette, cigarette lighter, clock, coaster, extension cord, eyeglasses, feather, film, flashbulb, flashlight, golf ball, hanger, keys, lightbulb, magnet, matches, nails, paint, picture frame, piece of wood, pillow case, pipe, radio, record, rocks, rope, screw, shoe polish, small mirror, small plant, small scale, sports equipment, stick or twig, string, tennis ball, thumbtack, vase, watering can, wire

Paper items: book, calendar, greeting card, magazine, map, napkin, newspaper, paper bag, paper towel, postcard, telephone book, tissue, toilet paper

Sewing items: buttons, crochet hook, elastic, embroidery frame, knitting needle, pieces of fabric, safety pin, tape measure, thread, yarn, zipper

Tools: chisel, drill, file, hammer, pliers, screwdriver, tin snips, wrenches

PICTURES OF OBJECTS

The following are examples of the pictures of objects you can use in the activities. They can be of any type so long as only one thing is shown in each picture. It is helpful to cut each of them out so you can use them again. The pictures should be easy to identify and should have no writing on them. Color pictures are preferable, but drawings of objects in black and white are fine too.

Advertisements: Newspapers (regular pages, ads in supplements, magazine sections, TV guides), magazines, special advertisements

Advertising circulars: Any type from a store, sent in the mail, added to newspapers or magazines, handed out door to door, or given out at special sales

Books: Photography books, art books, cookbooks (or recipes with pictures), other illustrated books

Children's books: Children's dictionaries, alphabet books, coloring books, and learning-to-read books found in drugstores, bookstores, libraries, book sections of department stores, toy stores, etc.

Catalogs: Mail-order catalogs for merchandise, department stores, gifts, foods, jewelry, clothing, crafts, gardening needs, and discount merchandise

Coupons: Those illustrating a product

Flyers, brochures: Similar to advertising circulars, either delivered free or found in public places

Junk mail: This comes in all types

Packages from foods and other products: Any picture of an item that you can cut out and use

Photographs of objects: In newspapers, magazines, photography or illustrated books, encyclopedias

ACTION PICTURES

The following are suggestions as to where to find pictures showing some action, a scene, or something happening.

Books: Any illustrated books, such as "how-to" or "fix-it" books, art books, travel books, books of photography, and children's books

Brochures, flyers: For resorts, tourist attractions, clubs or organizations, special products

Calendars: Calendars with pictures

Covers on boxed jigsaw puzzles

Covers on record albums, books, magazines, etc.

Magazines: Many popular, news, sports, and entertainment magazines

Newspapers: Pictures in the magazine supplements, comic strips, or special sections

Photographs: Family photo albums

Picture postcards

Posters: Travel, art, and decorative posters

LETTER TILES

If you own a game of Scrabble or something similar, the game's letter tiles can be used for the activities. If you do not, you can make your own tiles with unlined paper, a felt-tip pen, and scissors. (Cardboard or heavy paper is even better.)

Print the alphabet in capital letters on the paper. Each letter should be one-half to one inch high. Leave enough space between, above, and below each of the letters so they can be cut out separately. Print each of the letters A E I O U S R T two more times. Cut out each letter individually in a square shape. You should have forty-two letter tiles. Make more letter tiles if necessary.

Susan Howell Brubaker is Coordinator of Aphasia Rehabilitation in the Speech and Language Pathology Department of William Beaumont Hospital, Royal Oak, Michigan. She holds a B.S. degree from St. Lawrence University, Canton, New York, and an M.S. degree from Ithaca College, Ithaca, New York. She has earned the Certificate of Clinical Competence in Speech-Language Pathology from the American Speech-Language-Hearing Association. She is the author of *Workbook for Aphasia*, published in 1978.

This manuscript was edited by Harry Waldman. The book was designed by Betty Hanson. The typeface for the text is Baskerville, based on an original design by John Baskerville in the 18th century, and the display face is Univers. The paper is 60-lb. Arbor text paper. The book is bound in Riegel's Carolina CIS paper cover. Manufactured in the United States of America.

Suggestion Form

Your ideas will make this a better and more useful sourcebook. It would be helpful to know of any resources not listed in this book. If you are willing to share your information with others, please fill out the form below and send it to the address listed. If you are sending information about more than one item, please use additional sheets.

Indicate by a check mark what your information is about.

_____ book, pamphlet, or article about aphasia (include author)

_____ book, pamphlet, or article about some other helpful topic (include author)

_____ activity or game for more than one player (include manufacturer)

_____ activity or game to do alone (include manufacturer)

_____ information or reference from which you received help (indicate type of help and official name of source)

_____ other

Please explain as much about your source as possible.

_____

_____

_____

Please send your information and comments to:
Susan Howell Brubaker
Speech and Language Pathology Dept.
William Beaumont Hospital
3601 West 13 Mile Rd.
Royal Oak, Michigan 48072

Order Form

*Sourcebook for Aphasia: A Guide to Family
Activities and Community Resources*

Please send me_____copies of *Workbook for Aphasia* @ $10.95

_____ **Wulf,** *Aphasia, My World Alone* @ $9.50

_____ **Knox,** *Portrait of Aphasia* @ $7.95

_____ *SOURCEBOOK FOR APHASIA* @ $12.00

Name_____

Institution_____

Address_____

City_____State_____Zip_____

_____ Check or money order enclosed. Add $1.00 for postage and
handling.

_____ Please charge to my Mastercard ☐ or VISA ☐

Acct. No. ....

Bank No. (M/C) _____ Exp. Date _____

Michigan residents add 4% sales tax.